Transfusion Medicine

Blood Centre Methodology

Advance Techniques of Blood Components Preparation

Transfusion Medicine

Blood Centre Methodology

Advance Techniques of Blood Components Preparation

Bibekananda Mukherjee
BSc, DMLT (WHO-Fellow, Transfusion Medicine)
National Institute of Immunohaematology, ICMR, Mumbai
Senior Technologist
Department of Transfusion Medicine
Bokaro General Hospital, SAIL, Bokaro
Jharkhand

Gopal Krushna Ray
MD (Transfusion Medicine)
Assistant Professor
Department of Transfusion Medicine
All India Institute of Medical Sciences, Guwahati

CBSPD

CBS Publishers & Distributors Pvt Ltd

New Delhi • Bengaluru • Chennai • Kochi • Kolkata • Lucknow • Mumbai
Gujarat • Hyderabad • Jharkhand • Nagpur • Patna • Pune • Uttarakhand

Disclaimer

Science and technology are constantly changing fields. New research and experience broaden the scope of information and knowledge. The authors have tried their best in giving information available to them while preparing the material for this book. Although, all efforts have been made to ensure optimum accuracy of the material, yet it is quite possible some errors might have been left uncorrected. The publisher, printer and the authors will not be held responsible for any inadvertent errors or inaccuracies.

Transfusion Medicine

Blood Centre Methodology

Advance Techniques of Blood Components Preparation

ISBN: 978-93-49057-74-6

First Edition: 2025

Published by **Satish Kumar Jain** and produced by **Varun Jain** for

CBS Publishers & Distributors Pvt Ltd

4819/XI Prahlad Street, 24 Ansari Road, Daryaganj, New Delhi 110 002, India
Ph: 011-23266838, 23289259 Website: www.cbspd.com
e-mail: delhi@cbspd.com

Corporate Office: 204 FIE, Industrial Area, Patparganj, Delhi 110 092, India
Ph: 011-49344934 Fax: 011-49344935 e-mail: publishing@cbspd.com; publicity@cbspd.com

Branches

- **Bengaluru:** Seema House 2975, 17th Cross, KR Road, Banasankari 2nd Stage, Bengaluru 560 070, Karnataka, India
  Ph: +91-80-26771678/79 Fax: +91-80-26771680 e-mail: bangalore@cbspd.com
- **Chennai:** 18/8B, Subbarayan Street, Shenoy Nagar, Chennai 600 030, Tamil Nadu, India
  Ph: +91-44-42032115, 26681266 e-mail: chennai@cbspd.com
- **Kochi:** 42/1325, 1326, Power House Road, Opposite KSEB, Power House, Ernakulum 682018, Kochi, Kerala, India
  Ph: +91-484-4059061–65 Fax: +91-484-4059065 e-mail: kochi@cbspd.com
- **Kolkata:** 147, Hind Ceramics Compound, 1st Floor, Nilgunj Road, Belghoria, Kolkata 700056, West Bengal, India
  Ph: +91-33-25330055/56 e-mail: kolkata@cbspd.com
- **Lucknow:** Basement, Khushuma Complex, 7 Meerabai Marg (behind Jawahar Bhawan), Lucknow 226001, UP, India
  Ph: +91-522-4000032 e-mail: tiwari.lucknow@cbspd.com
- **Mumbai:** PWD Shed, Gala No. 25/26, Ramchandra Bhatt Marg, Next JJ Hospital, Gate No. 2, Opp. Union Bank of India, Noorbaug Mumbai 400009, Maharashtra, India
  Ph: +91-22-66661880/89 e-mail: mumbai@cbspd.com

Representatives

- **Gujarat** 0-9879558667
- **Hyderabad** 0-9885175004
- **Jharkhand** 0-9811541605
- **Nagpur** 0-8692091830
- **Patna** 0-9334159340
- **Pune** 0-9664372571
- **Uttarakhand** 0-9716462459

Printed at: HT Media Ltd, Greater Noida, UP, India

to

---

my respected honorable
Prof (Dr) Kanjaksha Ghosh
Prof (Dr) Sudipta Sekhar Das
Scientist Dr (Mrs) K Vasantha
Whose inspirations encourage and
support me, for good work

— Bibekananda Mukherjee

Foreword

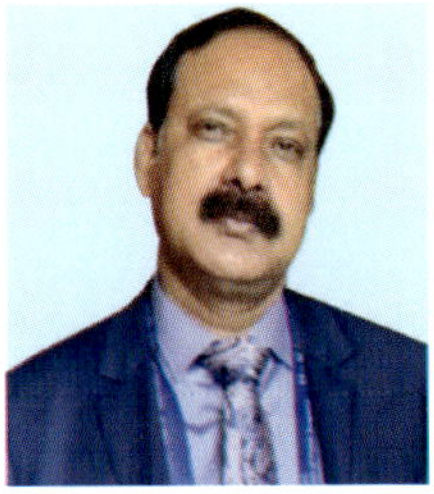

As the Executive Director of All India Institute of Medical Sciences, Guwahati, it is my distinct pleasure to introduce *Transfusion Medicine: Blood Centre Methodology and Advance Techniques of Blood Components Preparation*, authored by Mr Bibekananda Mukherjee and Dr Gopal Krushna Ray. This book is a significant contribution to the field of transfusion medicine and serves as an essential resource for healthcare professionals, educators, and students alike.

In the dynamic landscape of healthcare, the role of blood centers is critical. They not only ensure the safe and effective delivery of blood products but also uphold the highest standards of patient care. The authors have crafted a comprehensive guide that navigates the intricacies of immunohematology, detailing essential processes such as blood group serology, crossmatching techniques, and the management of complex cases like autoimmune hemolytic anemia (AIHA).

What sets this book apart is its practical approach. The authors emphasize the application of theory to real-world scenarios, offering detailed insights into techniques such as the Coombs test and the preparation of reconstituted blood for transfusions. Furthermore, the exploration of recent updates in donor selection criteria and blood component modification reflects the evolving nature of our field, ensuring that readers are well-informed of contemporary practices and innovations.

The meticulous attention to quality control, biosafety, and the management of biomedical waste highlights the authors' commitment to promoting safe practices in blood centers. This is increasingly vital in our quest to provide the highest quality of care and to safeguard the well-being of both donors and recipients.

As we strive to enhance the standards of transfusion medicine, this book will undoubtedly serve as a valuable reference. It encapsulates the essence of rigorous scientific inquiry and the practical application of knowledge, making it a pivotal addition to our educational resources.

I wholeheartedly commend Mr Mukherjee and Dr Ray for their remarkable work and invite all stakeholders in the field of transfusion medicine to engage with this insightful text.

Dr Ashok Puranik
Executive Director
All India Institute of Medical Sciences
Guwahati

Foreword

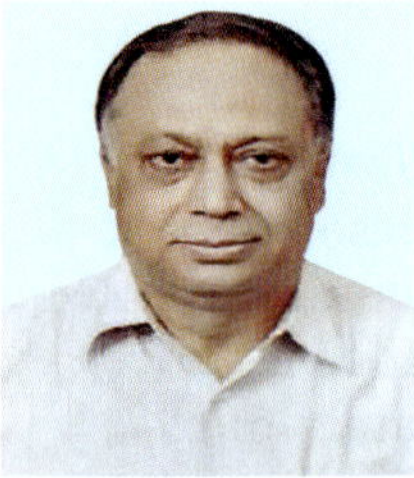

It gives me great pleasure to write the Foreword to this *Transfusion Medicine: Blood Centre Methodology and Advance Techniques of Blood Components Preparation* of Mr Bibekananda Mukherjee and Dr Gopal Krushna Ray.

Blood banking now called transfusion medicine has now flowered into a huge subject spanning not only basic blood bank operation but also apheresis technology, patient management, stem cell and many different types of cell cryopreservation and use for therapy. Production of tailor made cellular products for specific therapy, disaster management, management science, good manufacturing practice and so on.

However, this book is written for a specific purpose, i.e. to help the technical staff in the blood banking with ready reference for day to day work.

There has been increase in automation and molecular techniques have come up and slowly being taken up in advanced transfusion services.

However in India we have many small and medium sized blood banks both as standalone types and as a part in a medical college or a hospital. So we still need to have techniques which make technicians self-reliant, confident and capable of solving day to day problems within the limitations of cost, reagent, machinery and manpower.

This book will go a long way to fulfil this gap in the subject. The author also described some of the machines and advanced techniques which are used in blood banking.

Having several decades of experience in running a big blood bank and being trained in various techniques in some of the best centres in India, the author not only has the technical knowledge but also an insight and understanding the requirements of technicians in such a blood bank. He has produced an extremely useful book both for day-to-day work and those who wants to prepare for the examination in blood group serology.

I wish the author could have given names of some good reference books at the end of this manual which interested readers could consult. Few blank charts for antibody detection and a chapter on maintenance of various instruments, i.e. refrigerators, centrifuges, sealers, etc. would improve this manual.

Finally I consider this book to be an important addition in transfusion medicine manual in our country and will be received by all sections of the readers very well. I wish it much success.

Prof Kanjaksha Ghosh
MD (Med), DNB (Haem), MRCP (Ire), FRCPath (Lond), FRCP (Glasg), FACP (USA), FAMS, FICP, FNASc
Ex-Director
National Institute of Immunohaematology (ICMR) and
Ex-Hon Professor
Clinical Haematology and Transfusion Medicine
KEM Hospital, Mumbai

Foreword

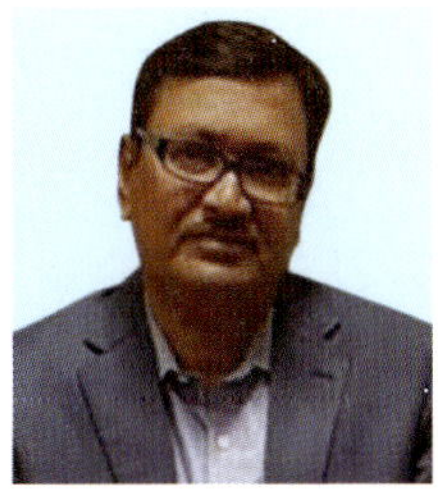

It gives me great pleasure to write the Foreword to this book *Transfusion Medicine: Blood Centre Methodology and Advance Techniques of Blood Components Preparation*. This is a convenient resource that has described not only the different methods of immunohematology or red cell serology but also the methods for blood component preparation. The book addresses major areas of transfusion medicine such as selection of donors, safe handling of equipment, calibration, preparation of components, component storage, component thawing, issue of component, transfusion doses, quality control, etc. It also gives an overview of methods in red cell serology and updates on recent technologies and techniques. This book meets the ready references for safe and qualitative preparation of blood components. It will be a useful reference for technologists working in advanced blood centres and for the transfusion medicine consultants.

Prof Rajendra Choudhary MD FRCPath
Former Professor and Head
Transfusion Medicine
SGPGIMS, Lucknow

Foreword

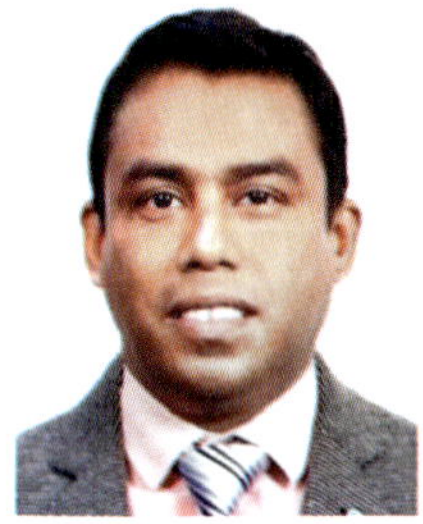

It gives me immense pleasure to mention the effort of Mr Bibekananda Mukherjee who besides his busy working schedule managed to prepare this book *Transfusion Medicine: Blood Center Methodology and Advance Techniques of Blood Components Preparation.* Mr Mukherjee who is currently the Senior Technologist in the Department of Transfusion Medicine and Blood Centre at the Bokaro General Hospital, Jharkhand, has put his hard work and very well enumerated his technical skill and experience in this practical book. I believe this book will enable the professional of transfusion medicine and blood centres to update their knowledge of blood bank laboratory methodologies and immunohematology.

Sudipta Sekhar das

Dr Sudipta Sekhar Das

Professor and Head

Department of Transfusion Medicine and Blood Centre

Apollo Multispeciality Hospitals, Kolkata

Sudipta.sgpgi@yahoo.co.in

Foreword

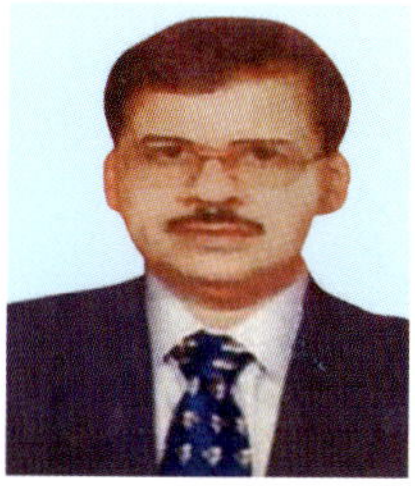

I am happy to learn that Mr Bibekananda Mukherjee, Senior Technologist, Department of Transfusion Medicine, Bokaro General Hospital, SAIL, Bokaro, Jharkhand, has prepared a laboratory manual entitled *Transfusion Medicine: Blood Center Methodology and Advance Techniques of Blood Components Preparation*.

Mr Mukherjee has been working in this center for more than 30 years. He attended a comprehensive training programme in blood banking which was organized for blood bank medical officers and technicians. National Institute of Immunohematology (ICMR) has been conducting this programme for more than 40 years and Mr Mukherjee was a participant of 2007 batch. He was sincere and hard working during this entire programme. He worked enthusiastically.

After completing this programme, he started thinking that whatever I learned here should be compiled and put forward in the form of a book. He started working on that and finally the idea is materialized.

This book tells us about overview of blood bank set up, basic immunohematology, blood grouping techniques. It also tells us about some advanced techniques like resolution of blood group discrepancies, absorption elution test, secretor status test, etc. Preparation of sensitized cells, crossmatching techniques, use of ELISA in blood bank, evaluation of transfusion reaction are also mentioned in this book. Finally the component therapy which is the important aspect in modern blood banking is also explained here.

This book will be useful to all the medical officers and technicians working in blood bank in the remote area, and also to those who are newcomers in the field of transfusion medicine or immunohematology.

I congratulate Mr Bibekananda Mukherjee for his tireless efforts in bringing out this laboratory manual.

Dr Ajit C Gorakshakar

Former Scientist (Senior Deputy Director)
Former Head, Department of Transfusion Medicine
ICMR-National Institute of Immunohaematology
Indian Council of Medical Research
13th Floor, New Multi Storeyed Bldg
KEM Hospital Campus, Parel
Mumbai 400012, India

Preface

Modern medical science has undergone rapid progress due to advancements in technology. Transfusion medicine plays a pivotal role in life-saving situations. Nowadays, many advanced technologies are used for the collection of human blood, testing, and component preparation in a blood centre. In today's life, human blood is transfused in several ways and acts as medicine for treating a number of diseases.

It is an immense pleasure for us to write this book ***Transfusion Medicine:*** *Blood Centre Methodology and Advance Techniques of Blood Components Preparation*. With our vast technical experience, we feel basic knowledge about blood centre is required for those who are sincerely engaged in this profession. We have included the basic concept of immunohematology and blood component preparation. The testing methods of immunohematology through the conventional tube technique are properly described, including proper washing, accurate temperature and time of incubation, speed (rotation per minute), proper cell suspension preparation and proper ratio of serum/plasma and cell suspension.

The blood components should be prepared with utmost care towards quality. Adequate precautions are to be followed throughout the transfusion chain, starting from the collection, testing, component preparation, processing, storage, and compatibility testing. Advanced techniques of blood component preparation through automated machines have been described in this book. Very few centers have the facility for apheresis. The technical tips given here are for the smooth running of apheresis and the steps for troubleshooting.

We have made our best efforts to present practical knowledge related to routine procedures in a blood centre, written in a simple and easily understandable language.

The book is particularly intended for the medical laboratory technicians, undergraduate and postgraduate students of medical laboratory technology and paramedical courses, technicians working in blood centres, and MBBS students who wish to learn various aspects of blood centre methodology.

Bibekananda Mukherjee
Gopal Krushna Ray

Acknowledgments

I am very much indebted to honorable Prof (Dr) Kanjaksha Ghosh, former Director, NIIH (ICMR), Mumbai, and Hon. Professor, Department of Hematology, KEM Hospital (Mumbai), who always motivates me for good work. It is my good luck that I have received a fellowship award from that great person.

It is my immense pleasure that I have dedicated the book to the renowned person of medical fraternity in India. I believe that he acted like a godfather to me as he recommended my hard work. I feel that it is one of my life-time achievement award to get recognition from such a laurel personality.

I am indebted to honorable Prof (Dr) Utpal Chaudhuri, former Director, IHTM, Medical College, Kolkata, for his valuable recommendation regarding my previous published components preparation book.

I am especially indebted to the honorable Prof (Dr) Sudipta Sekhar Das, Head of the Department of Transfusion Medicine, Apollo Multispecialty Hospital, Kolkata, who always encourages and supports me for good work and also delivers me up-to-date knowledge of blood centre methodology and immunohematology. Dr Das always welcomes the people of medical fraternity with open arms and his heartfelt help always plays a vital role in accomplishing the project of people like us.

I am indebted to the honorable Dr Bipalabendu Talukdar, Professor, Department of Immunohaematology and Blood Transfusion (IHBT), Kolkata Medical College and Hospital, Kolkata, who always encourage and support me for good work.

I am indebted to the honorable Dr (Mrs) K Vasantha, Former Scientist, NIIH (ICMR), Mumbai, who always paid special attention to me while teaching blood centre methodology and blood centre serology during fellowship training. Her valuable guidance/training has proven to be milestone for trainees across the country.

I am indebted to the honorable Dr (Mrs) Swati Kulkarni, Scientist, NIIH (ICMR), Mumbai. Who always encourage and support me for good work.

I am indebted to the honorable Dr Ajit C Gorakshakar, former Scientist, NIIH (ICMR), Mumbai. His contributions in NIIH (ICMR) has helped the people of medical fraternity especially the persons who are working in blood centres. His valuable guidance has helped me to acquire new ideas about blood centres during fellowship training.

I am also indebted to the honorable Dr Pruthvi Raj Guduri, Head, Department of Transfusion Medicine, The Mission Hospital, Durgapur, for guiding me properly with constant support to complete this work. I feel enthralled to get his prompt suggestions throughout this project.

I am very much grateful to Mrs Seema Yadhav, NIIH (ICMR), Mumbai, who gave me a lot of practical tips during the training period.

I express my gratitude to my respected elder brother late Mr Swapan Kumar Mukhopadhyay. It is my pride that such an academician and honest person's cooperation and love I got since my childhood. I want to give my heartfelt gratitude to my elder brother for his continuous support.

I express my thanks to beloved Mrs Anjali Mukherjee for her valuable inputs (both technical and academic) and helping and co-operating me during rain or shine in the whole journey of my book's preparation.

My beloved daughter Dr Deepshikha Mukherjee and nephew Dr Indranil Chakraborty, constantly supported and shared their updated knowledge for completing the manuscript.

I express my gratitude to honorable senior doctors in Bokaro General Hospital, SAIL, and honorable senior professors from different medical colleges who always motivates me for good work and always inspired me since the beginning of my career. I would like to thank Dr Bibhuti Bhushan Karunamay, Director, Dr Anand Kumar, Director, Dr Aninda Mandal, Director, Dr Upendra Mohanty, Dr Prasanta Kumar Sarkar, Dr Thounaojam Momon Singh, Dr S K Sinha, Dr Abhijit Dam, Dr Aniruddhra Bandyopadhyay, Dr (Mrs) Chandreyi Bandyopadhayay, Dr Indranil Choudhary, Dr Anil Agarwal, Dr Devendra Kumar, Dr Nilay Pathak, Dr Vijay Chandra Jha, Dr Saket Mishra and Dr Trinath Panchal. Prof (Dr) Prasun Bhattacharya (Transfusion Medicine-Medical College Kolkata, Prof (Dr) Somnath Mukherjee, Transfusion Medicine, AIIMS, Bhubaneshwar, Prof (Dr) Malay Ghosh, Transfusion Medicine, RBTC, RG Kar Medical College, Kolkata.

I wish to thank all technologist those working in Department of Transfusion Medicine who have helped in the preparation of this technical manuscript and expressed their ideas regarding this book.

Mr Sanjay Kumar, Mr Mahendra Prasad, Mr Manish Patrick and Mr Mosesh P Hembram (Bokaro General Hospital, SAIL), Mr Avijit Pal (RSP Hospital, SAIL), Md Safi (Appolo Hospital, Kolkata), Mr Samipendu Mukherjee (Mission Hospital, Durgapur), Mr Ashutosh Jha (Technical Superviser, Shrinivas Blood Centre, Hazaribagh). Mr Abhishek Dhar (Jamshedpur Blood Centre).

I also want to acknowledge those persons who always support me from time to time during the completion of this work. Dr Sagar Chatterjee (Ortho Diagnostic), Mr Waman Keshav Narkar (NIIH, ICMR), Mumbai, Mr Jayanta Roy Chaudhary (Bio-Rad Diagnostic), Mr Animesh Mukherjee (Rose Diagnostic), Mr Sanjay Choudhary (Jamshedpur Blood Centre, Jamshedpur), Mr Rajarshi Mukherjee (Nephew), Mrs Mithu Banejee (Baro-didi), Mrs Jharna Mukherjee (Baudi), Mrs Reena Sarkar (Baudi), Mr Kaushal Kr Jha, Mr Pradip Kumar Ghoshal and my dear best friend Mr Ghanshyam Sharma.

I am for ever thankful and deeply indebted to my parents late Smt. Shankari Mukherjee and late Shri Noni Gopal Mukherjee for the love and grace bestowed upon me. I canot forget my departed beloved brother late Shri Ramkrishna Mukherjee whose immeasurable affection inspired me to accomplish this noble work.

Bibekananda Mukherjee

Contents

PART II: Advance Techniques of Blood Components Preparation

Abbreviations

Ab	Antibody
ACCL/DECL	Acceleration/deceleration
ACD	Acid-citrate cextrose
Ag	Antigen
AHF	Antihemophilic factor
AHG	Antihuman globulin
AHTR	Acute hemolytic transfusion reaction
AIHA	Autoimmunohaemolytic Anemia
BBR	Blood bank refrigerator
BBRC	Blood bag refrigerated centrifuge
BC	Buffy-coat
BCNO	Blood centre number
BMW	Biomedical waste
BV	Blood volume
C	Centigrade
CAT	Column agglutination technique
CBC	Complete blood count
CP	Cryo-precipitate
CPCB	Central pollution control board
CPDA/CPD	Citrate phosphate dextrose adenine/citrate phosphate dextrose
CTT	Conventional tube technique
DAT/DCT	Direct antiglobulin test/direct Coomb's test
DHTR	Delayed haemolytic transfusion reaction
Du Test	Weak D test
DVET	Double volume exchange transfusion
EDTA	Ethylene diamine tetraacetic acid
ELISA	Enzyme linked immunosorbent assay
FFP	Fresh frozen plasma
FNHTR	Febrile nonhaemolytic transfusion reaction
HDFN/HDN	Hemolytic diesease of fetus and newborn/hemolytic dieases of newborn
Hrs	Hours

HTR	Haemolytic transfusion reaction
IAT/ICT	Indirect antigloubulin test/indirect Coombs test
LISS	Low-Ionic strength saline solution
PAS	Platelet additive solutions
PEP	Postexposure prophylaxis
PLTC/PL	Platelet concentrate/platelet
PPH	Postpartum hemorrhage
PPP	Platelet-poor plasma
PRP	Platelet-rich plasma
PRC/PRBC	Packed red cell/packed red blood cells
PTP	Posttransfusion purpura
RBC	Red blood cell
RCF	Relative centrifugal force
RDP	Random donor platelets
RPM	Rotation per minute
RT	Room temperature
SAGM	Saline adenine glucose mannitol
SDP	Single donor platelets
SOP	Standard operating procedure
TTI	Transfusion transmissible infection
TACO	Transfusion associated circulatory overload
TA-GVHD	Transfusion associated-graft vs host disease
TEMP	Temperature
TRALI	Transfusion related acute lung injury
UV	Ultraviolet
VDRL	Venereal disease research laboratory
VOL	Volume
WBC	White blood cell

PART

I

Blood Centre Methodology

Chapter 1

Overview of Blood Centre

The **blood centre** has basically six different working areas apart from the store-cum-record room, such as

a. Donor complex (rooms for donor counseling, medical examination, blood collection, refreshment, apheresis)
b. Serology lab (immunohematology)
c. Serology lab (transfusion transmitted disease screening)
d. Component separation lab
e. Quality control lab
f. Sterilization-cum-washing room

All the working areas should be well-lightened, and ventilated with air-conditioning. The equipment or reagents required in these concerned laboratories are as follows:

a. Donor complex

1. Blood donor couch
2. Bio-mixture or blood collection monitor
3. Hemoglobin estimation (HemoCue or any equipment that measurs Hb quantitatively)
4. Sphygmomanometer and stethoscope
5. Weighing machine
6. Lancet/Needle
7. Vacutainer (EDTA and plain)
8. Blood bag (single, double, triple, quadruple, inline-filter: Top and top or top and bottom)
9. Desktop and Barcode printer
10. Tube sealer
11. Apheresis machine
12. Transportation box
13. Blood bank refrigerator 2 to 6°C.
14. Domestic refrigerator
15. O_2 cylinder
16. Crash cart (emergency medicine)
17. Emesis basin

b. Serology lab (immunohematology)

1. Test tubes: Standard glass test tubes (Kahn tube 10 mm × 80 mm/pilot tube 12 mm × 100 mm), precipitin test tubes 10 mm × 50 mm, or conventional tube technique (CTT), standard test tubes 12 mm × 75 mm, or 10 mm × 75 mm (whatever is available), Microprecipitin test tubes (5 mm × 50 mm), use for micro-volume.
2. Test tube rack
3. Antisera (anti-A, anti-B, anti-D, antihuman globulin (AHG), anti-IgG, anti-C3d)
4. Lectin (anti-A1, anti-H)
5. Column agglutination technology (Gel card-blood grouping, Coombs card, neutral card, monospecific card)
6. Gel card incubator and centrifuge
7. Table top centrifuge (*see* Fig. 3.1)
8. Micropipette
9. Pasture pipette/disposable dropper
10. Incubator
11. Serological water bath
12. Advanced immunohematology antisera and other reagents
    - Minor antisera (Rh, Kell, Duffy, Kidd, MNS, Lewis, Lutheran)
    - Low ionic strength salt solution (LISS), phosphate buffer solution, HCl,
    - Antibody screening panel (2-cell/3-cell panel)
    - Antibody identification panel (11-cell panel, 16-cell panel)
    - Elukit (glycine-HCl)
    - Adsorption [(polyethylene glycol (PEG)], albumin
    - Enzyme (ficin, papain, L-cysteine)
13. Glass slides
14. Wash bottle, beakers, conical flask, and measuring cylinder
15. Binocular microscope
16. Automated immunohematology analyzer

c. Serology lab (transfusion transmitted disease screening)

1. ELISA washer and reader (semi- or fully-automated)
2. Micropipette
3. VDRL-shaker
4. ELISA plate, buffer, control (negative and positive), enzyme, stopper for HIV-1,2, HBV, HCV, malaria
5. ELISA wash buffer, container
6. Chemiluminescence analyzer
7. Nucleic acid amplification test (mini pool or ID-NAT)

d. Component separation lab

1. Double pan weighing scale
2. Refrigerated blood bag centrifuge
3. Laminar air flow
4. Plasma expressor
5. Stand for blood bag hanging

6. Weighing scale
7. Blood bank refrigerator
8. Deep freezer (–80°C, –40°C)
9. Platelet incubator-cum-agitator
10. Cryo-bath
11. Plasma thawing bath
12. Sterile connective device
13. Blast freezer
14. Automated component extractor
15. Tube sealer and tube stripper
16. Automated blood component processor (Reveos®)

e. Quality control lab

1. Hematology analyzer (CBC analyzer)
2. Coagulometer (semi or fully-automated)
3. pH meter
4. Negeotte chamber
5. Thromboelastogram (TEG/ROTEM®)
6. Platelet function analyzer
7. Timer and stopwatch

f. Sterilization room

1. Autoclave
2. Hot-air-oven

All the areas of a blood centre should be equipped with the biomedical waste bins, disposable waste bags, hypochlorite solution, Hazmat spill kit, etc. as per the BMW management rules.

The following forms and registers are required for the smooth functioning of a blood centre:

1. Donor form (bilingual donor questionnaire)
2. Blood requisition form
3. Compatibility form
4. Transfusion reaction reporting form
5. Color code label
6. Adverse donor reaction reporting form (register)
7. Donor register
8. Donor deferral register
9. Rare donor register
10. Cross-match register
11. Issue register
12. Blood group register
13. Component preparation register
14. Master register
15. TTI screening register
16. Discard register
17. Stock register
18. Log book for each equipment

Chapter 2

Immunohematology and Blood Group Serology

INTRODUCTION

The basic concept of immunohematology and blood group serology is based on antigen and antibody reactions. A proper ratio of plasma or serum to red cells is essential to attend the zone of equivalence where the maximum strength of antigen–antibody reactions is achieved. Too heavy a concentration of either serum or cells might cause a weak or false negative reaction, i.e. prozone or post-zone phenomenon. Patients with abnormal albumin-to-globulin ratios may cause pseudoagglutination (rouleaux), so adequate washing is important during the red cell suspension preparation. EDTA vial (violet top) is used for the detection of red blood cell antigens and a clot-activated vial (red top) is for the presence of antibodies in the serum.

DEFINITION OF ANTIGEN AND ANTIBODY

Antigen: Antigen is any substance which on introduction into a human body, stimulates the production of a specific antibody and reacts with that specific antibody in an observable manner. Most commonly, it is a protein or polysaccharide.

Antibody: Antibody is a substance that is produced in serum or tissues on the introduction of specific foreign antigens and reacts with that antigen in an observable manner. Chemical nature of antibody = Immunoglobulin.

Result: Antigen (RBC) + Antibody (serum/plasma) = Agglutination.

Prozone Phenomenon

The phenomenon means when specific antigens and antibodies are mixed, it does not agglutinate or precipitate visibly because of the presence of excess antibodies. It means the test is incorrect or unsuccessful.

Classification of antigen and types of antigen reaction:

1. Complete antigen.
2. Incomplete antigen or haptens antigen.

   Haptens antigen are two types:

   a. Complex haptens.

   b. Simple haptens.

a. **Complete antigen:** A substance that is sufficient to stimulate the production of antibodies and also binds to the antibody.

b. **Incomplete antigen/haptens antigen:** A substance that only can stimulate the production of antibodies after the attachment of a carrier protein.

> ***Example:*** A hapten is essentially an incomplete antigen.

Classification of antibodies and types of antibody reaction:

1. According to physiochemical and antigenic differences properties.
   Classes of antibodies are:

   IgG, IgA, IgM, IgD, and IgE

   IgM and IgG are the important antibodies in the field of immunohematology.
2. According to thermal activity of the reacting temperature:
   i. Warm antibody.
   ii. Cold antibody.
3. According to visible reaction (Fig. 2.1).
   1. Complete antibody.
   2. Incomplete antibody.

Warm antibody: An antibody that reacts with the corresponding antigen at 37°C is called a warm antibody.

IgG is a warm antibody.

Cold antibody: Antibody which reacts with the corresponding antigen at cold (0–4°C) or room temperature is called a cold antibody.

IgM is a cold antibody.

Complete antibody: Antibody which reacts with the corresponding antigen and gives visible reaction agglutination in the saline phase (immediate spin); is called a complete antibody (as shown in Fig. 2.1).

> ***Example:*** IgM antibody is a complete antibody as it is a pentavalent antibody.

Anti-A and anti-B are IgM type antibody (natural occurring).

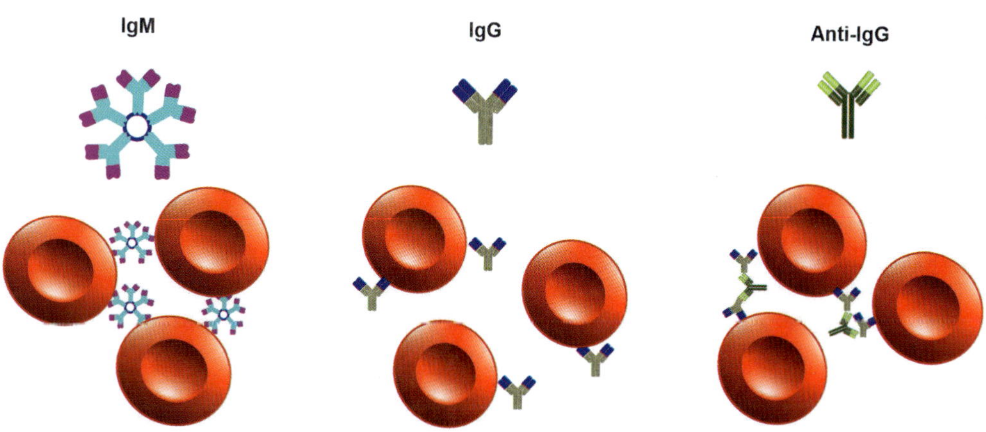

Fig. 2.1: Example of complete and incomplete antibody

Incomplete antibody: Antibody that reacts with the corresponding antigen but does not produce a visible reaction (sensitized RBC) is known as incomplete antibody. It requires antihuman globulin (AHG) to show visible agglutination (AHG phase).

> ***Example:*** IgG is an incomplete antibody. Because it is a bivalent antibody that coats the red cells when incubated at 37°C, but does not show visible agglutination. It is known as sensitization. With the help of AHG, agglutination the red cells formed.

FACTORS AFFECTING ANTIGEN–ANTIBODY REACTION

- Temperature
- pH
- Ionic strength
- Enzyme treatment of red cells
- Concentrations of antigen and antibody
- Zygosity (number of antigen sites per cell—homozygous or heterozygous)
- Duration of incubation

For proper antigen and antibody reaction, adequate precautions are to be taken as follows:

- Conventional tube technique (CTT) or column agglutination (CAT) is to be used in serology testing. Do not practice the glass slide technique in blood centre serological testing.
- Precipitin test tube (10 mm × 50 mm), recommended standard glass test tube (12 mm × 75 mm) or micro-precipitin test tube (5 mm × 50 mm) is used in the blood centre for serology testing in CTT method, as antigen and antibody reaction occurs properly.
- Some manufacturer's make standard serological glass test tubes (10 mm × 75 mm) and it can be used also in blood centre serological testing in CTT method.
- If the volume of the sample (serum/red blood cell suspension) is less then use micro-precipitin test tube.
- Plastic tubes or plastic-coated glass tubes should not be used for any serological test because the result of the test is not clearly visible.
- Use Kahn/pilot tube or commercially available barcode vacationer (12 mm × 100 mm) for blood sample collection.
- Use a pilot tube for red blood washing and red blood cell suspension preparation.
- Do not use Kahn or pilot tubes (12 mm × 100 mm) for blood centre serological testing.
- Serum is preferred over plasma for different testing in immunohematology because it is free from fibrin clots.
- Always fresh samples are preferred and never use the haemolysed samples (serum/cells) for blood centre serological test.
- Ratio of serum to cells—for proper antigen–antibody reaction (binding) we have to maintain the zone of equivalence by taking two parts of serum and one part prepared 2–5% of red blood cells suspension (preferred 5% of red blood cell suspension in normal saline) (ratio 2 in 1) for reverse grouping, cross-matching and antibody screening/detection by conventional tube technique (CTT) as per AABB guidelines.

- Ratio of serum to cells—equal volume of serum and prepared 2–3% of red blood cell suspension in low ionic strength saline (LISS) is used (ratio 1 in 1) for blood grouping in gel card.
- During testing, carefully place the serum/plasma, red blood cells, and antisera at the bottom of the tube, and then mix them gently. Do not touch the inner surface of the tube, serum/red cell suspension will remain attched on the wall of the test tube and sufficient mixing during incubation may not happen.
- During testing, hold the pasture pipette or micropipette in a vertical position for respective collection of serum, reagent, antisera and prepare red blood cells suspension, etc. and put at 180° angle inside the serological test tubes and mix gently without bubbles formation.
- During testing, use the same gauge pasture pipette for the respective collection of serum, normal saline, antisera, reagents, red blood cells suspension, etc. because the ratio of volume should be equal.
- Always use standard clean glass pipette and glass pasture pipette with rubber tit (borocil/corning).
- The tip of the pasture pipette should not be broken.
- Glassware must be cleaned, detergent-free and dry during testing.
- Fixed pipette and variable micropipette should be calibrated.
- Take out test kits with antisera, reagents, prepared red blood cells suspension, and sensitized red cells (Coombs control cell) from the blood bank refrigerator and keep them on the working table for a minimum of 30 minutes before starting the test.
- Strictly follow the time of incubation, check the temperature of the incubator, proper washing of the red blood cells, rpm, and timing of centrifugation according to the instruction of blood centre SOP (standard operative procedure) and the machine should be calibrated in CTT method.
- Temperature—IgM antibodies react optimally at or below 22°C whereas IgG reacts best at 37°C.
- The washing of red blood cells is used to remove the protein (globulin) which might cause false agglutination.

Chapter 3

Saline-washed Red Blood Cells and Pooled Red Blood Cells Suspension

PREPARATION OF CELL SUSPENSION AND ITS USE

The ABO blood group system is characterized by the presence of an 'A' or 'B' antigen on the red blood cells. To detect the antibody, present in the plasma/serum of a patient or donor, a known antigen is required. The donor red cell whose blood group has already been confirmed, is the commonly used source of antigen. Red cells from three to five different donors of the same ABO group are pooled to prepare a red cell suspension. This helps to have a greater expression of antigens and better detection of antibodies. 'A' cell, 'B' cell, and 'O' cell are prepared daily from known A, B, and O blood group donors for routine blood group serology. In a blood centre, 5% cell suspension is used for tests performed by CTT and 0.8–1% cell suspension for CAT.

Preparation of Red Blood Cell Suspension

Materials Required

- Test tube
- Test tube rack
- Normal saline (0.9%)
- Red blood cell (donor cell)
- Table top centrifuge
- Micropipette or pasture pipette

Preparation of 1%, 2%, 3%, and 5% saline wash red blood cell suspension for blood grouping, cross-matching (IgM and IgG), Du and DAT test.

Red blood cell washing and cell suspension preparation procedure:

Method:

- Take pilot test tubes (12 mm × 100 mm) and mark on tubes with a marker for the donor, recipient, or individual test (like blood group, Rh typing, cross-matching, and Du test. Takes several drops of blood (8–10 drops for 5% or 4–6 drops for 2% or 3% red blood cells) from the fresh anti-coagulated blood sample (EDTA/CPD/CPDA).
- Fill approximately three-fourths level of the tube with normal saline (0.9%) and mix well.
- Centrifuge with 'high spin' at 3500 to 4000 rpm for 3–5 minutes, until red blood cells are settled at the bottom of the test tube. (Try putting RCF values as RPMs change from centrifuge to centrifuge).
- Remove the test tube from the centrifuge machine after stopping the centrifuge.

- Decant the supernatant fluid from tubes as much as possible.
- Remove any debris or fibrin with the clean pipette.
- Repeat this process 3–6 times (minimum three times), till the supernatant fluid becomes clear.
- Decant the supernatant fluid from tubes as much as possible.
- Red blood cells are washed to remove the plasma proteins, unbound antibodies or Warton's jelly (newborn) which may interfere in the blood group serology.
- Take another pilot test tube and prepare 1%, 2%, 3% or, 5% of red blood cell suspension as per requirement.
- For preparing 1% of red blood cells suspension, take 10 µl of packed red blood cells from washed RBC and 990 µl of normal saline (0.9%) or 1 drop of packed red blood cells from washed RBC and 99 drops of normal saline using standard pasture pipette and mix well.
- For preparing 2% of red blood cells suspension, take 20 µl of packed red blood cells from washed RBC and 980 µl (0.9%) of normal saline or 2 drops of packed red blood cells from washed RBC and 98 drops of normal saline using standard pasture pipette and mix well.
- For preparing 5% of red blood cells suspension, take 50 µl of packed red blood cells from washed RBC and 950 µl (0.9%) of normal saline or one drop of packed red blood cells from washed RBC and 19 drops of normal saline using standard clean pasture pipette and mix well.

Preparation of Red Cell Suspension of Patient

- Follow the same procedure to prepare red blood cell suspension of the particular donor or patient sample for blood grouping, Coombs test, cross-matching, etc.
- Always prepare a fresh red blood cell suspension before performing any of the tests in blood group serology.
- Always use the donor blood bag segment for preparing suspension for blood grouping and cross matching tests (donor red blood cell).

USE OF 2%, 3%, AND 5% SALINE-WASHED RED BLOOD CELLS SUSPENSION

- Red blood cell suspension is used for:
  - Blood grouping, Rh typing, and Du testing (Patients)
  - Direct antiglobulin test (DAT)
  - Cross-matching (donor red cell)
- Red blood cell suspension (2–5%) is used for blood grouping, Rh typing, and Du testing. (Washing of red blood cell must be practiced, especially in every newborn baby, cold antibody, mother cord blood and others discrepancies.)
- Prefer 5% of red blood cell suspension for serological tube testing.
- **Cross-matching:** 2% to 5% of red blood cells suspension is used for saline and enzyme cross-matching (prefer 5% of cells suspension for serological tube testing).
- Prefer 5% of red blood cell suspension for IAT cross-matching.
- Always follow the instructions of the blood centre SOP.

Preparation of 2%, 5%, 10% and 50% 'A1', 'A2', 'B' and 'O' blood group pooled red blood cells suspension and its use.

Use of pooled red blood cell suspension in blood centre serology:

Pooled red blood cells are prepared by taking 3–5 different red blood cells unit to get adequate different types of antigenic expression. All minor antigens like Kell, Kidd, Duffy, MNS are present in different proportion on red cell surface, so to get almost all antigens we make pool cells. The pooled red blood cells are used for reverse grouping, IAT, antibody detection, sensitized red blood cell preparation, and titration of the antisera.

Method

- Take four pilot test tubes (12 mm × 100 mm) and mark on the tubes with a marker for the desired saline washed pooled red blood cells suspension like 'A$_1$' cell, 'A$_2$' cell, 'B' cell and 'O' cell.
  For example: Select a minimum 3–5 confirmed donors having individual 'A$_1$' blood group red blood cell and prepare daily from fresh samples.
- Take 2–5 ml of blood from freshly anticoagulated 'A$_1$' blood group red blood cell unit either whole blood or the prepared packed red blood cell (PRBC).
- Apply this process to 'A$_2$', 'B' and 'O' blood group tubes also.
- Wash the red blood cells 3–4 times in a large volume of normal saline. Centrifugation at 3,500–4,000 RPM (try putting RCF values as RPMs change from centrifuge to centrifuge) for 3–5 minutes.
- Decant the supernatant fluid from tubes as much as possible.
- Follow the instruction above mentioned steps about washing.
- Take separate four pilot test tubes (12 mm × 100 mm) and prepare 2%, 5%, and 50% of pooled red blood cells suspension for 'A$_1$', 'A$_2$', 'B' and 'O' blood group according to the requirement (Table 3.1).
- For preparing 2% of pooled red blood cell suspension, take 20 µl of pooled packed red blood cells from saline washed RBC tube and 980 µl (0.9%) of normal saline or 2 drops pooled packed red blood cells and 98 drops of normal saline using standard pasture pipette and mix well.
- For preparing 5% of pooled red blood cells suspension, take 50 µl of pooled packed red cells from saline washed RBC tube and 950 µl (0.9%) of normal or take one drop pooled packed red blood cells from saline washed RBC tube and 19 drops of normal saline using standard glass pasture pipette and mix well. The color of red blood cell suspension looks like ripe red tomato.

Table 3.1: Cell suspension preparation

Preparation of red blood cells suspension	1%	2%	3%	4%	5%
Packed red blood cells volume, ml	The final volume, diluted with saline, in ml				
0.1 ml = 100 µl of PRBC	990 µl N/S + 10 µl PRBC	980 µl N/S + 20 µl PRBC	970 µl N/S + 30 µl PRBC	960 µl N/S + 40 µl PRBC	950 µl N/S + 50 µl PRBC
1 ml = 1000 µl of PRBC	0.99 ml N/S + 0.01 ml PRBC	0.98 ml N/S + 0.02 ml PRBC	0.97 ml N/S + 0.03 ml PRBC	0.96 ml N/S + 0.04 ml PRBC	0.95 ml N/S + 0.05 ml PRBC

- For preparing 10% of pooled red blood cells suspension, take 100 µl of pooled packed red blood cells from saline washed RBC tube and 900 µl (0.9%) of normal saline or 10 drops pooled packed red blood cells and 90 drops of normal saline using standard pasture pipette and mix well.
- For preparing 50% of pooled red blood cells suspension, take 100 µl of pooled packed red blood cells from saline washed RBC tube and 100 µl (0.9%) of normal saline or 50 drops pooled packed red blood cells and 50 drops of normal saline using standard pasture pipette and mix well.
- Prepare fresh pooled red blood cells suspension daily before starting the test.
- Pooled red blood cells suspension should be used within 12 hours of preparation (prefer 8 hours) and keep the prepared above red blood cells suspension in blood centre refrigerator at 2–6°C temperature until it is used.
- Do not use the haemolysed pooled red blood cells suspension for blood centre routine test and any serological test.

Use of 2–3%, 5% and 50% confirm 'A_1', 'A_2', 'B', and 'O' blood group rh positive or negative pooled saline wash red blood cells suspension:

Pooled red blood cell suspension (A cell, B cell, O cell) is used for

Reverse grouping

- A cell and B cell are used to detect anti-A, anti-B, respectively.
- 'A_1', 'A_2' and 'B' blood group Rh-positive pooled red blood cells suspension is used for reverse grouping (prefer 5%). Sometimes, A_2 cells are required in reverse grouping to resolve blood group discrepancy due to anti-A1 in a patient or donor of A (A_2) blood group.
- 'O' group pooled red blood cells suspension (prefer 5%) is used for screening test of irregular unknown antibody detection (allo-antibodies) present in the plasma or serum through saline IgM and papin cysteine enzyme (IgG).
- 'O' group pooled red blood cells suspension (prefer 5%) is used to detect anti-H which is present in the plasma of Bombay blood group donor or patient (for screening test). If show agglutination, then confirm Bombay group by the presence of 'H' antigen utilizing anti-H lectin.
- Using 2–5% of 'O' group Rh-positive pooled red blood cells suspension for Rh-antibodies titer detection (saline IgM and enzyme IgG). Prefer 5% of red blood cells suspension for serological tube testing.

Indirect antiglobulin test (IAT)

- 'O' cell is used for IAT, as it lacks both 'A' and 'B' antigens. So, it will not interfere with the anti-A and anti-B of the patients.
- 'O' group Rh-positive and Rh-negative red blood cell are pooled to prepare the red blood cells suspension (prefer 5%) for IAT.
- 'O' positive R_1 R_1 (DCe/DCe) and 'O' negative rr (dce/dce) cells are taken for better antigenic expression. (A ratio of pooled is 3 in 1 (Three Rh +ve and One Rh –ve having individual) is preferred.
- Apart from Rh, to obtain a better expression of other minor blood group antigens like Kell, Duffy, Kidd, MNS, and Lutheran, pooled 'O' cell is used for IAT.

- Antibody screening is a type of IAT, where 'O' cell of known antigens with homozygous expression is used to get a preliminary idea on suspected antibodies. Commercially prepared two, or three or four cell panel is available. A suspected antibody can be identified by performing antibody identification (11-cell or 16-cell panel).
- Pooled 'O' blood group red blood cell suspension is prepared by taking pilot tubes (12 mm × 100 mm) from known 'O' blood group blood bags present in the inventory. Both of pooled red cells for IAT (IgG) and also used for reverse grouping (IgM) reaction.
- 'O' group Rh-positive pooled red blood cells suspension (prefer 5%) is used for the preparation of sensitized red cells (Coombs control cells) for validity check of the test IAT and DAT.

Titration of Antisera

- 5% of corresponding antigen containing pooled red blood cells suspension (blood group Rh +ve or Rh –ve) is used for titration of antisera checking.
- 'A' antigen pooled red blood cell (A_1, A_2, A_1B and A_2B) are used for antisera 'A' (IgM) titer.
- 'B' antigen pooled red blood cell (B, A_1B and A_2B) are used for antisera 'B' (IgM) titer.
- 'A' and 'B' antigen pooled red blood cells (A_1, A_2, A_1 B, A_2B and B) are used for antisera 'AB' (IgM) titer.
- 'O' blood group pooled red blood cells is used for antisera 'H' lectin titer.
- 'A_1' blood group pooled red blood cells suspension is used for antisera A_1 lectin titer.
- 'O' blood group Rh +ve pooled red blood cells suspension is used for antisera 'D' (IgM and IgG) titer.

Specificity of Antisera

- 2–5% of A_1, A_2, B, O, A_1 B and A_2B blood group, Rh +ve or Rh -ve pooled red blood cells suspension is used for checking-specificity of antisera for 'A', 'A'$_1$, 'B' and antisera 'AB' (prefer 5% of red cells suspension for serological tube testing, CTT).

Avidity of Antisera

- 50% of A_1, A_2, A_1B and A_2B blood group Rh +ve or Rh –ve antigen containing red blood cells suspension. It is used for checking the avidity of antisera 'A'.
- Similarly, B, A_1B and A_2B blood group Rh +ve or Rh –ve pooled red blood cells suspension are used for checking the avidity of antisera 'B'.
- A_1, A_2, A_1B, A_2B, and B group Rh +ve or Rh –ve pooled red blood cells suspension are used for checking the avidity of antisera 'AB' (50% of pooled red blood cells

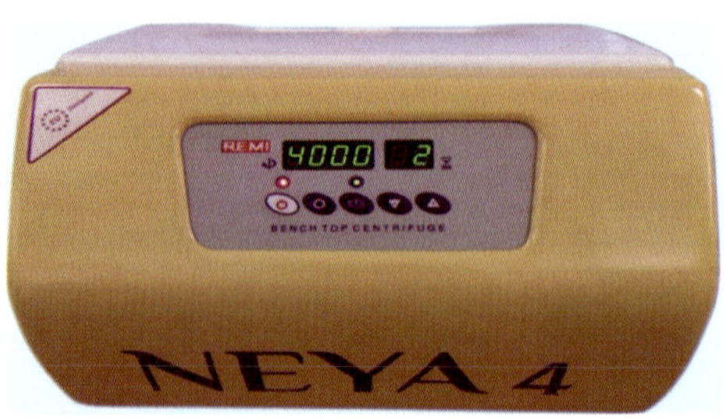

Fig. 3.1: Table top centrifuge (digital)

suspension is used as per DGHS guidelines), RhD positive pooled O cell suspension (50%) is used to test the avidity of anti-D.

Diluting an Existing Dilution

1. A new higher dilution can be prepared from diluted material by adding more diluent. The formula for calculating either the new higher final dilution or the amount of diluents to add to obtain a higher final dilution is:

$$\frac{\text{Reciprocal of present serum dilution}}{\text{Volume of serum dilution used}} = \frac{\text{Reciprocal of new final dilution}}{\text{Total final volume}}$$

2. **Example:** Serum dilution is one in two and volume of serum dilution is 1.0 ml. If 4.0 ml of saline is added, what will be the new final dilution?

$$2/1 = X/5$$

$X = 10$ or 1 in 10 dilutions.

Method: Dilution of % solutions.

Procedure

Dilutions can be prepared from more concentrated solutions by use of the following formula:

$$\text{Volume}_1 \times \text{Concentration}_1 = \text{Volume}_2 \times \text{Concentration}_2$$

$$V_1 \times C_1 = V_2 \times C_2$$

where, V_1 and $C_1 = V_2 \times C_2$ represent original volume and concentration, and V_2 and C_2 represent final desired volume and concentration.

Chapter 4

ABO and Rh Blood Group System

BLOOD GROUPING TECHNIQUE, ANTISERA, LECTIN AND OTHER USEFUL REAGENTS AND THEIR USES

Blood Grouping Antisera, Lectin and Other Reagents Used in Blood Centre

- In general blood centering practice three antisera are used for blood grouping.
- Anti 'A'
- Anti 'B'
- Anti 'D' (monoclonal-IgM)
- Extra antisera are used in special conditions (Fig 4.1a).
- **Anti-AB:** For confirmation of presence of subgroups of 'A' or 'B' antigen in case of blood group discrepancy (weak antigen expression).
- **Anti-A_1' lectin *(Dolichos biflorus)*:** For subgroup classification of 'A' and 'AB' subgroup ('A_1', 'A_2' and 'A_1B', 'A_2 B')
- **Anti-'H' lectin *(Ulex europeas)*:** For detection of Bombay phenotype and secretor status studies through saliva.
- **Anti-'D' blend (IgG + IgM):** Used for routine RhD detection and weak D (Du) test of RhD negative donor unit.

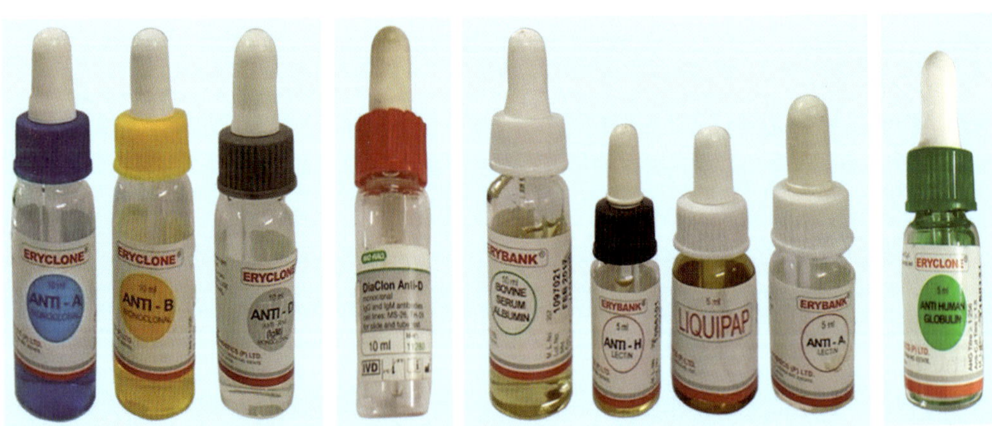

Fig. 4.1a: Blood grouping antisera, lectin and other useful reagents

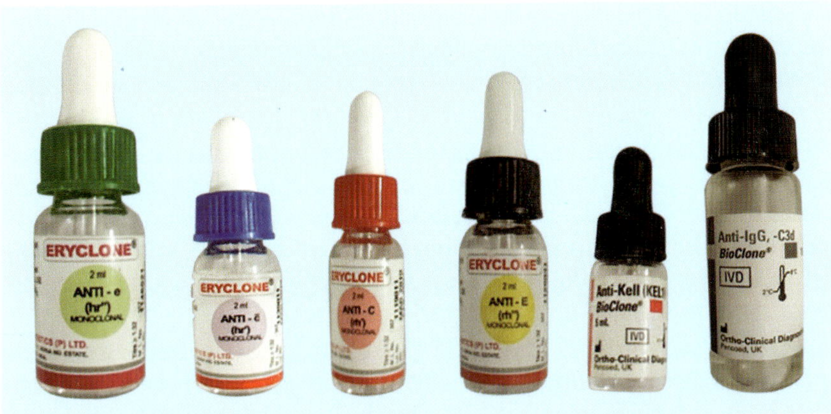

Fig. 4.1b: Minor antisera (anti-e, anti-c, anti-C, anti-E, anti-K) and AHG

- **Anti-'D' monoclonal (IgG):** Used for Du test to confirm D variants, and as a positive control for IAT test and sensitize red cells preparation.
  1. **NB:** If anti-'D' (IgG) commercially is not available, blend (IgG + IgM) anti-'D' can be used for Du test.
  2. **Uses of minor antisera:** The anti-C, anti-E, anti-c, anti-e and anti-K reagents detect the presence of antigens C, E, c, e and K on the surface of red blood cells (Fig. 4.1b).
- **Uses of sensitized red blood cells (Coombs control cells):** To check the validity of DAT and IAT.
- **Uses of papain cysteine reagent:** Enzyme cross-match and to identify the antibodies where multiple alloantibodies are suspected (one is enzyme sensitive and other one is enzyme resistant).
- **Uses of 6% of bovine albumin reagent:** For IgG cross-matching and absorption studies using bovine albumin.
- **Uses of antihuman globulin (AHG) reagent:** For IAT cross-matching, IAT, DAT, Rh antibody detection test, and IAT control.
- **Monospecific AHG (anti-IgG, anti-C_3d) are used in tube test:** Antihuman globulin (anti-IgG and anti-C_3d) is use to detect sensitized RBC (either coated with IgG or C_3d).
- **Use of LISS solution:** LISS is used as a potentiator. It increases the rate of antibody uptake and therefore decreases the incubation time. It is also used for column agglutination technique (Gel card method) and absorption studies.
- Always use two different manufacturer's antisera for blood grouping and Rh (D) typing test which is mandatory according to drug control norm. Always follow the instruction of the blood centre SOP.

ABO Blood Group Systems

The ABO Antigens and Corresponding Antibodies

The red cell membrane carries various types of surface proteins, and proteins that cross the lipid layer of the cell membrane. These surface proteins and glycoproteins carry the blood group antigens and their specificity is mostly determined by the sequence of oligosaccharides (e.g. ABO) or the sequence of amino acids (e.g. Kell, Duffy, Kidd, MNS). These antigens are assigned to blood group systems or collections based on their relationship to each other as determined by serological or genetic studies. As of November 2023, the red cell Immunogenetics and blood group terminology working party of the International Society of Blood Transfusion (ISBT) recognised 45 blood group system genes containing 362 antigens. In this chapter, the basics of ABO blood group system, and the methods of blood grouping will be discussed.

The ABO antigens and antibodies are the most important for blood transfusion service. It is the only blood group system in which the reciprocal antibodies are consistently and predictably present in the sera of most people, without any previous exposure to human red cells. Transfusion of ABO-incompatible blood may cause severe intravascular hemolysis due to this natural occurring antibody.

Genes at three separate loci (H, Se, and ABO) control the occurrence and the location of the A and B antigens. H gene is responsible for the synthesis of H antigen from which 'A' or 'B' or both or none is produced. As per the synthesis of ABH antigen, the ABO blood group is defined (Fig. 4.2 and Table 4.1).

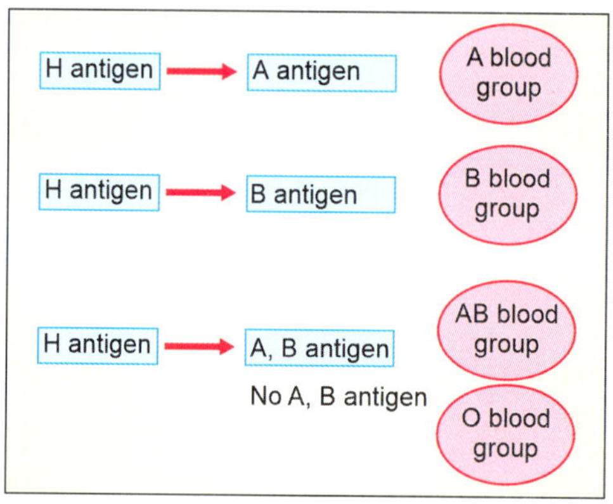

Fig. 4.2: The ABO antigens and corresponding antibodies

Table 4.1: ABO blood group antigens and their corresponding antibodies

Antigen on red cell surface	*Antibody in plasma/serum*	*Blood group*
A	Anti-B	A
B	Anti-A	B
A, B	None	AB
H (No A or B Ag)	Anti-A , Anti-B	O
—No H, A, B Ag	Anti-A, Anti B, Anti-H	Bombay

'O' blood group has anti 'A' and anti 'B' antibodies but no antigen.
'B' blood group has 'B' antigen and anti 'A' antibody.
'A' blood group has 'A' antigen and anti 'B' antibody.
'AB' blood group has 'A' and 'B' antigens but no antibody.

BLOOD GROUPING AND RH TYPING TEST OF UNKNOWN CELLS

- **Blood group:** Genetically determined antigen system.
- Expressed mostly on the RBC surface and it can be detected by potent (efficient) antisera.

Rh Blood Group System

Two highly homologous genes on the short arm of chromosome 1 encode the non-glycosylated polypeptides that express the Rh antigens. These genes are RHD and RHCE which produce 57 antigens. Among these Rh antigens, D, C, c, E, e; are more important. RhD antigen is clinically most significant and its presence is termed as RhD positive and its absence as RhD negative.

Blood Grouping by CTT

Materials/Reagents Required

- Test tube
- Test tube rack
- Table top centrifuge
- Normal saline
- Anti 'A'
- Anti 'B'
- Anti 'D' (monoclonal-IgM)
- Anti D (blend IgG + IgM)
- Anti-AB
- Anti-H
- "A" cell, "B" cell, and "O" cell

Methodology

1. *Forward grouping (cell grouping):*
   a. The principle is agglutination of unknown antigen by known antibodies (commercially available antisera). (Cell/Forward/Direct grouping is based on an agglutination reaction between A- and B-antigen present on RBCs which agglutinates with commercial anti-A and anti-B antisera, respectively.
   b. Blood group A is further divided into A_1 and A_2 based on this, the ABO blood group system can be divided into six subtypes group A_1, A_2, B, A_1B, A_2B and O.
   c. Only forward grouping (cell grouping) is to be done for newborns baby till 4 months of age.

2. *Reverse grouping (serum grouping):*

It is the principle of detection of anti-A and anti-B present in the plasma or serum by using pooled red blood cell suspension.

Procedure

- Take standard glass test tubes, labelled it properly and arrange serially from left-to-right direction according to the mark in a test tube rack.
- The wooden rack has been already marked 'A', 'B', 'D1' and 'D2' (Rh) for cells grouping, 'A_1'cells, 'B' cells,'O' cells, for serum grouping (Fig. 4.3).
- Mark sample number on all tubes by marker.

- Prefer fresh samples for testing and do not use the haemolysed serum and haemolysed red blood cells suspension for blood group serology.
- Take two drops (or 100 µl) of respected antisera 'A', 'B', 'D1' and 'D2' (IgM) according to the labelled test tubes.
- Collect unknown test serum (donor/recipient) using pasture pipette or micropipette and place two drops (or 100 µl) in serum grouping in each tube.
- Add one drop (or 50 µl) of prepared 2–5% of red blood cell suspension using clean pasture pipette or micropipette for cells grouping in each tube (prefer 5% of red blood cells suspension for CTT).
- Add 5% 'A_1' cells, 'B' cells, and 'O' cells for reverse grouping in the respective test tubes (Table 4.2).

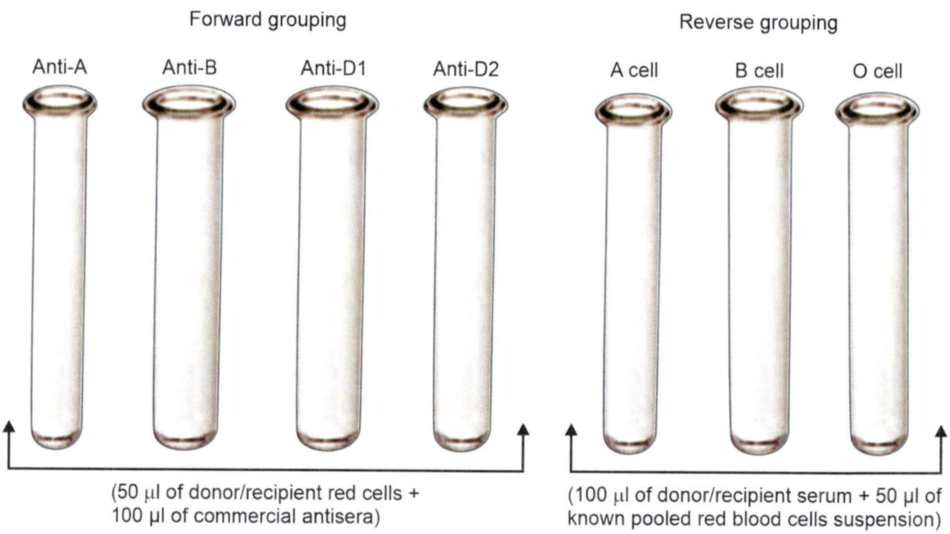

Fig. 4.3: Blood grouping technique through tube method

Table 4.2: Cell grouping and reverse grouping

Cell grouping (Antisera monoclonal)				*Serum/reverse grouping (Antibody screening, donor/recipient)*			
Anti-A	*Anti-B*	*Anti-D1*	*Anti-D2*	*A cell*	*B cell*	*O cell*	*Blood group*
+	0	+	+	0	+	0	A RhD +ve
0	+	+	+	+	0	0	B RhD +ve
+	+	+	+	0	0	0	AB RhD +ve
0	0	+	+	+	+	0	O RhD +ve
0	0	+	+	+	+	+	Bombay RhD +ve*
+	0	0	0	0	+	0	A RhD –ve
0	+	0	0	+	0	0	B RhD –ve
+	+	0	0	0	0	0	AB RhD –ve
0	0	0	0	+	+	0	O RhD –ve

*Agglutination with O cell in reverse grouping warants to test the red cell with anti-H lectin to confirm Bombay (oh) blood group.

INTERPRETATION

Conventional tube technique (CTT) is shown in Fig. 4.4.

Writing for result graded as follows (Fig. 4.4):

++++ Complete single clump.
+++ Several large clumps.
++ Medium size clumps, clear background.
+ Multiple small clumps, turbid background.
+w Weak agglutination.
–Ve (Negative) No clump.

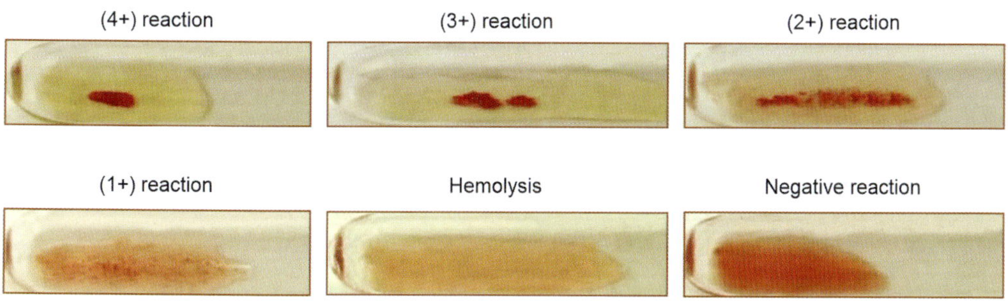

Fig. 4.4: Agglutination grading in conventional tube technique (CTT)

NB: Tubes are centrifuged to enhance the antigen–antibody binding.

Column Agglutination Technique

There are two kinds of methods which are applied for the column agglutination technique. They are:

1. Glass microbeads method
2. Gel card method

1. COLUMN AGGLUTINATION TECHNIQUE BY GLASS MICROBEADS METHOD

Principle

Reis KJ had described the above technique/system for irregular antibodies in the year 1993. The above-mentioned test is performed in a microcolumn prefilled with glass microbeads in the suspension of antihuman globulin serum, any diagnostic reagent, or neutral isotonic solution. During column centrifugation, the sensitized cells are trapped by the microbeads suspension. Detection of sensitized red cells is based upon the sieving effect of glass microbeads. At the upper part of a column over the glass microbeads suspension, red cells, and serum are incubated. During the centrifugation step they retain the agglutinations and the unsensitized cells settles at the bottom.

The follow materials are required for the process:

- BioVue cassettes.
- BioVue centrifuge.
- BioVue incubator.

- BioVue system work rack.
- BioVue liner.
- Micropipettes 10 µl, 40 µl and 50 µl.

Cell suspension preparation for glass micor-beads method:

- **Preparation of 4% red cell suspension:** Take 960 µl of normal saline in a standard test tube and 40 µl of packed RBC of A/B/O cells
- Mix gently to make cell suspension homogenous.

Red blood cell suspensions preparation as per requirement using isotonic saline and packed red blood cells.

Normal saline	*Packed red blood cell volume*	*Red blood cell concentration %*
970 µl	30 µl	3%
960 µl	40 µl	4%
950 µl	50 µl	5%
1.2 ml	10 µl	0.8%
990 µl	10 µl	1.0%

Forward Grouping and Reverse Grouping by Glass Microbeads Method

- Prepare red blood cell suspension
- Allow the cassette to come to room temperature before use.
- Open the wells of the cassette using the liner assembly (Fig. 4.5a).
- The cassette should be used within one hour after insertion of the liner.
- **For forward grouping:** Add 10 µl of 3% to 5% or 40 µl of 1.0% or 50 µl of 0.8% red blood cell suspension to the reaction chambers of the cassette (columns 1, 2, 3, and 4) (Fig. 4.5b).
- **For reverse grouping:** Add 50 µl of 0.8% or 10 µl of 3% pooled cell to the appropriate reaction chambers of the cassette (column 5 and 6).
- Add 40 µl of serum/plasma to the appropriate reaction chambers of the cassette (column 5 and 6).
- Centrifuge the cassette using the BioVue system centrifuge.
- Centrifuge should occur within 30 minutes of addition of the samples to the reaction chamber.
- Read the front and back of the individual columns for agglutination and/or hemolysis upon test completion.

The following are some of the advantages of using glass microbeads technique:

- The incubation period/time is as low 10 minutes for antibody screening or cross-matching.
- Approximately, 5 minutes time for biphasic centrifugation.
- There is no need to wash cells or use sensitized cells for confirmation in AHG test
- There is no tube shaking or re-suspension of cells button leading to variation in reading and grading the agglutination.

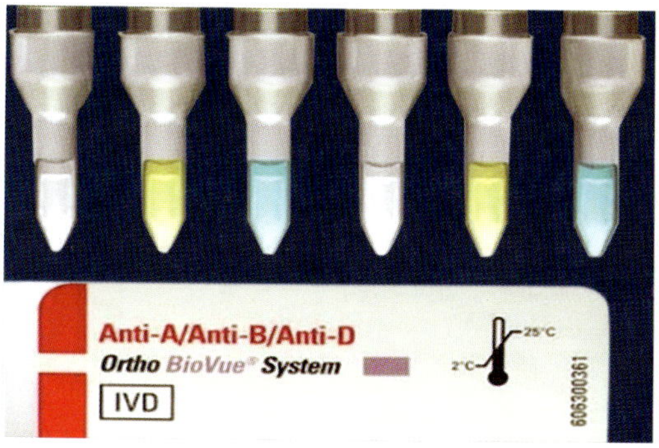

Fig. 4.5a: ABO forward grouping card

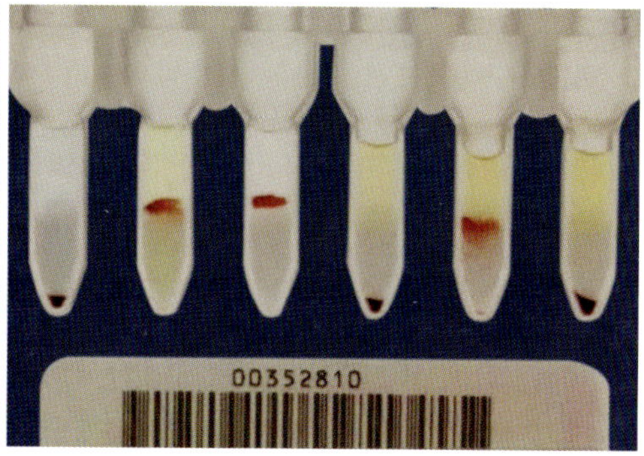

Fig. 4.5b: ABO forward and reverse grouping card

- Due to the provision of a calibrated centrifuge to spin at the optimal speed for a fixed and correct length of time, the margin of error during this phase of the test is less.
- The interpretation of the result is more objective, consistent, and reproducible.

Protocol for Coombs Test (DAT/ DCT) by Glass Microbeads Method in Ortho BioVue System

Preparation of 4% red blood cell suspension:

Add 50 µl of packed RBC cell of test sample (washed once in saline) in 1.0 ml (1000 µl) of normal saline solution and mix gently.

Procedure:

- Open the aluminum foil of the BioVue casstte.
- Add 10 µl of 3–5% RBC suspension.
- Centrifuge the cassette for 5 minutes using BioVue centrifuge.
- Read the result.

Indirect Coombs Test (ICT) by Glass Microbeads Method in Ortho BioVue System

Procedure:

- Centrifuge the sample supplied at 3000 rpm for 3 minutes to get supernatant test serum.
- Open the aluminum foil of the BioVue cassette.
- Add 50 µl LISS reaction chamber.
- Add 10 µl of 3–5% pooled 'O' red cell suspension.
- Add 40 µl of test serum.
- Incubate at 37°C for 10 minutes OWS incubator.
- Centrifuge the cassette for 5 minutes using BioVue centrifuge.
- Read the result.

2. COLUMN AGGLUTINATION TECHNIQUE BY GEL CARD METHOD

- For column agglutination technique (CAT), please follow the manufacturers instruction.
- Red blood cell suspension of 0.8 to 1% is used in CAT testing (whereas 5% cell suspension is used in CTT) and dispensed into the reaction chamber by micropipette at an angle of 45°.
- Serum is dispensed by the micropipette at perpendicular to the gel card.

- Blood grouping, direct antiglobulin test (DAT) and indirect antiglobulin test (cross-matching, antibody screening/identification) can be performed by CAT method which is more sensitive compared to tube technique.
- In CAT, washing step is not required as the unbound antibody cannot interfere in the agglutination process like that of CTT.
- Serum or plasma can be used in (gel card method) column agglutination technique for reverse grouping, cross-matching, antibody screening, and indirect anti-globulin test. Centrifuge the anticoagulated (EDTA) sample and keep that plasma in a separate tube and this plasma is used for the above test. Serum is prefered for antibody screening as complement activating antibodies may be missed while using plasma for the test.
- Strictly follow the time of incubation, check the temperature of the incubator, rpm, and timing of centrifugation according to the manufactures instruction.
- During incubation, check that the incubator is maintaining the temperature at 37°C. Observe the result immediately after completing the test procedure.

BLOOD GROUPING AND REVERSE GROUPING BY COLUMN AGGLUTINATION TECHNIQUE (GEL CARD METHOD)

The gel column acts as a filter that taps agglutinated red blood cells as they pass through the column during the centrifugation of the card. The gel column separates agglutinated red blood cells from non-agglutinated red blood cells based on size.

Reagents/apparatus required:

- Gel card: ABO/D + Reverse grouping card.
- Test tubes (CTT).
- Micropipette.
- Gel card centrifuge machine.
- Gel card warmer (incubator).
- Prepared readymade diluents (LISS solution).
- A_1 cells, B cells, O cell (0.8 to 1% suspension), ready to use for reverse grouping.
- Donor and recipient red blood cells and serum/plasma.
- Tissue paper/cotton/normal saline/distill water.
- Gel card rack and test tube rack.

Instructions of gel card pipetting.

✓ **Right instructions:** Pipetting of red cells suspension at 45° angle and pipetting of serum at 90° angles (Figs 4.6a and b).

× **Wrong instructions:** Pipetting of red blood cells suspension and serum.

Red blood cell washing is not required for cell suspension preparation in the column agglutination technique (gel card method).

Step 1

- Preparation of 1% A,B, O cell suspension for reverse grouping and 5% test red cell suspension for forward grouping.
- Take 1000 µl of readymade diluents (LISS or NS) + 10 µl of donor packed RBCs in a precipitin tube. Take 950 µl LISS + 50 µl red cell (test sample) to prepare 5% cell suspension.

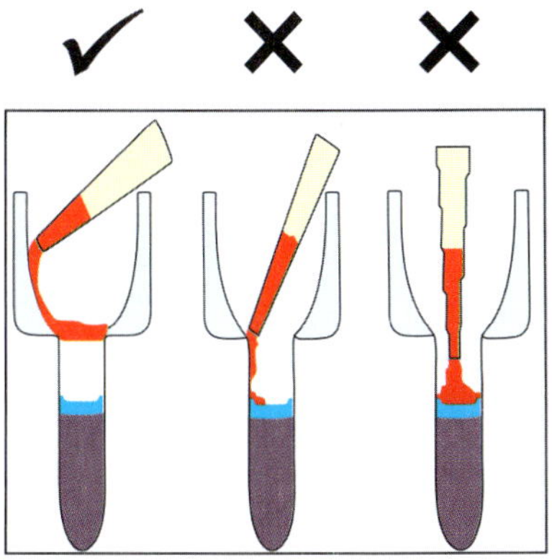

Fig. 4.6a: Pipetting of red ells

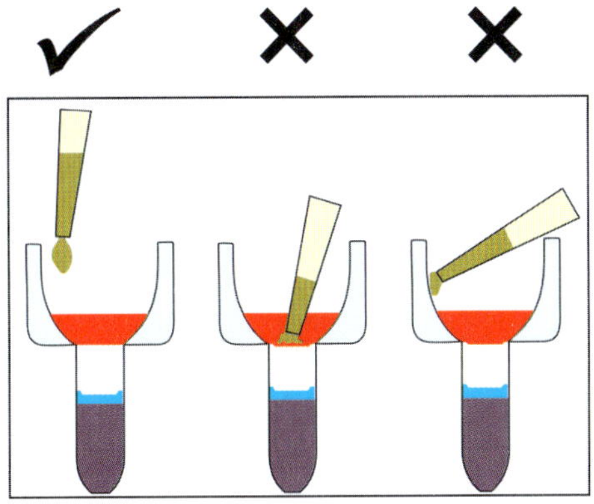

Fig. 4.6b: Pipetting of serum/plasma

Step 2

- Forward grouping.
- Remove aluminum foil of micro-tube in upright position of the card (Fig. 4.7a).
- Add 10–12.5 µl 5% cell suspension (test) red blood cells suspension of sample to be tested in gel micro-tube labelled as A, B, D.

Step 3

- Reverse grouping.
- Add 50 µl of readymade 'A_1' cell, B cells, and O cells to gel micro-tube labelled as A_1, B and O cell (control)
- Add 50 µl of serum/plasma (prefer serum) of sample to be tested in both gel micro-tube labelled as A_1, B and control.

Step 3

Incubate at room temperature for 10 minutes and then centrifugation for 10 minutes in gel centrifuge machine.

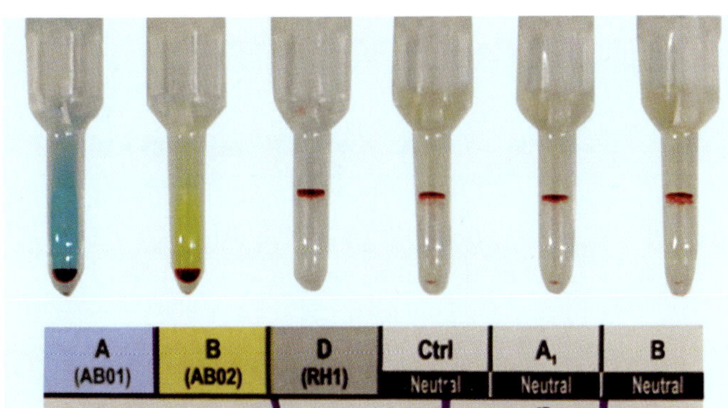

Fig. 4.7a: Blood grouping gel card (Bombay Rh postive)

Note: Details of Bombay blood group is discussed in Chapter 5.

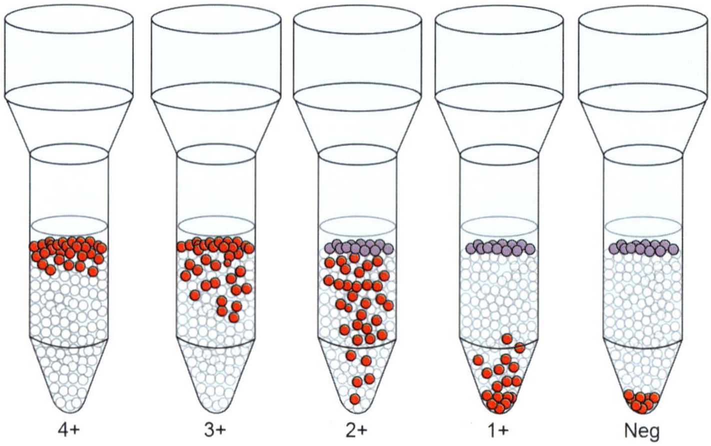

Fig. 4.7b: Grading of agglutination

Step 4

Read results and grades the result as mentioned in Fig. 4.7b.

The control test is always negative. If the control shows agglutination that indicates clot, contamination, or auto-agglutination of the sample.

Newborn Blood Grouping

Reagents/apparatus required

- ABD/Rh for newborn gel card (Fig. 4.8).
- Readymade diluent (LISS solution).

Follow the above mentioned blood grouping and an extra ABD/Rh newborn gel card is needed for newborn grouping. (Reason—newborn blood sample is cord blood sample containing Whartons jelly which may produce a false positive reaction.)

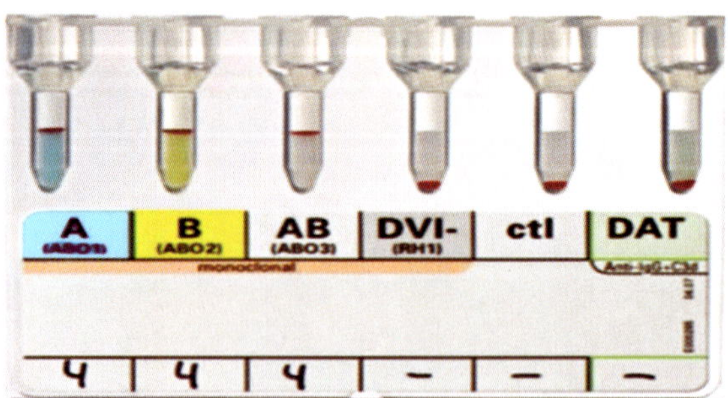

Fig. 4.8: Newborn grouping and DAT

Step 1

0.8–1% red blood cell suspension preparation.

Take 1000 µl of readymade diluents (LISS solution) + 10 µl of the newborn patient's packed RBCs in a precipitin tube. Mix gently.

Step 2

Forward grouping and DAT:

Remove the aluminum foil of the micro-tube in the upright position of the card.

Add 50 µl of the above-suspended cell to all 6 micro-tubes of gel card.

Step 3

Centrifugation for 10 minutes in a gel centrifuge machine.

Result interpritetion: Blood group is reported as per the agglutination observed in the gel cards.

Rh and Kell Subtyping by Column Agglutination Technique (Gel Card)

Reagents/apparatus required

Rh subgroup + Kell gel card (Fig. 4.9).

And follow the same above-mentioned blood grouping and an extra Rh subgroup + Kell gel card is needed for Rh and kell subtyping.

Step 1

5% red blood cell suspension preparation.

Take 500 µl of readymade diluents (LISS solution) + 25 µl of patients-packed RBCs in a precipitin tube. Mix gently.

Or

1% cell suspension:

Take 950 µl of readymade diluents (LISS solution) + 50 µl of patients-packed RBCs in a precipitin tube. Mix gently.

Step 2

Add 50 µl of above 1% red blood cell suspension of samples (10 µl of 5%) to be tested in a micro-tube labelled as C, c, E, e, Kell, and control.

Step 3

Centrifugation for 10 minutes in a gel-centrifuge machine.

Result interpritaion: Agglutination in the gel column is considered as positive and the Rh, Kell phenotype is reported accordingly.

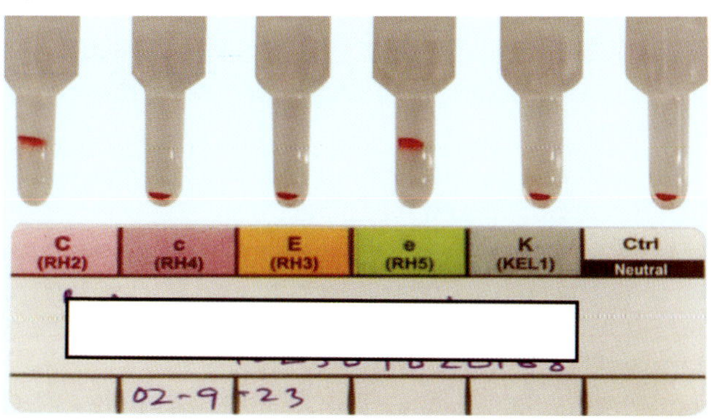

Fig. 4.9: Gel card for Rh subgroup and Kell

Chapter 5

Resolution of Blood Group Discrepancy

- ABO blood grouping can be performed by simple technique and it involves two basic steps—cell grouping (forward grouping) that establishes the presence or absence of A- and/or B-antigens on the red blood cells (RBCs) and serum grouping (reverse grouping) that demonstrates the presence or absence of ABO antibodies in the serum.
- Determination of the correct ABO blood group needs both cell grouping and serum grouping because of the existence of a mutual association between cell grouping and serum grouping.
- Blood group discrepancies are usually encountered when there is a deviation from the expected pattern of antigen in cell grouping and antibody in serum grouping. In other words, blood group discrepancy is the mismatch between the expected forward and reverse grouping.
- These blood group discrepancies occur due to weaker expression of A- or B-antigens or missing or low titer of ABO antibodies. Other reasons may be related to technical error or clerical error, miscellaneous, or rouleaux formation, which gives rise to the blood group discrepancy.
- As per the standard classification of ABO discrepancy, blood group discrepancy is divided into four major categories—type I, type II, type III, and type IV ABO blood group discrepancy

RESOLUTION STEPS FOR BLOOD GROUP DISCREPANCY

- Always ask for a fresh sample to repeat the blood group.
- Check for clerical error.
- Rule out wrong blood in the tube (WBIT means the blood inside the sample tube or vacutainer is of different patient and the name and registration number mentioned on the tube is different.)
- Usually, higher strength of agglutination is considered as true agglutination and the missing agglutination is considered for further test.
- If the blood group discrepancy is due to missing antibody in the plasma, then increase the serum to cell ratio that is four-part serum instead of two-part and one part cell. If still there is no agglutination, increase the duration of incubation or incubate the cell-serum mixture at 4°C, then check for agglutination.
- If the blood group discrepancy is due to missing antigen, then increase the cell to serum ratio that is one part serum and cell each. If still there is no agglutination,

Table 5.1: Types of ABO discrepancy and their causes

Type I	*Type II*	*Type III*	*Type IV*
Weak or missing antibodies	*Weak or missing antigen*	*Rouleaux formation*	*Miscellaneous or irregular antibody*
• Newborn • Elderly patients • Patient with leukemia or lymphoma • Patients on immunosuppressive drugs • Patients with immunodeficiency diseases • Patients with bone marrow transplant	• Subgroups of A or B • Leukaemia and lymphoma • Excess antigen of blood group soluble substances • Acquired A- or B-antigens and Hodgkin's lymphoma	• Elevated levels of plasma globulins: Multiple Myeloma, Waldenstrom's macroglobulinemia, and Hodgkin's lymphoma • Elevated levels of fibrinogen • Use of plasma expanders such as dextran • Wharton's jelly in cord blood samples	• Poly agglutination • Patient with cold autoantibodies • A_2 or A_2 B individual with anti-A_1 antibodies • Naturally occurring or irregular antibodies reacting at room temperature • Cis-AB (Cis-AB, a rare ABO variant, is caused by a gene mutation that results in a single glycosyltransferase enzyme with dual A and B glycosyltransferase activities)
RESOLUTION			
• Increase serum: Cell • Increase incubation time • Incubate at 4°C	• Increase cell: Serum • Increase incubation time • Incubate at 4°C	• Saline replacement technique is the established method to resolve rouleaux. (After centrifugation, remove the plasma and add equal volume of saline) Rouleaux will no longer be seen when the plasma proteins are removed.	• Monoclonal antisera and use of lectin • Poly-agglutination • Antibody screening/identification • Pre-warming technique • DTT treatment (Dithiothreitol) which breaks IgM antibody

increase the duration of incubation or incubate the cell-serum mixture at 4°C, then check for agglutination.

- Even then there is no agglutination is detected in both the types of discrepancy, elution-adsorption technique is performed.
- **Saline replacement technique:** This method is required when false agglutination is suspected in reverse grouping in a patient of multiple myeloma or paraproteinemia. Do the reverse grouping by CTT as described previously (Chapter 4). Do not check for agglutination. Rather, remove the supernatant plasma from all three test tube and add equal volume of normal saline. If there is true agglutination, it will remain as it is. But the false agglutination will disperse.
- **Pre-warming technique:** If the blood group discrepancy is due to a cold antibody, then keep the disposable syringe, needle, vacutainer, normal saline and pipette at 37°C. Immediately after collecting the sample, separate the plasma from cell. Keep the serum at 37°C for one hour and then repeat reverse grouping. Wash the cell with the warm saline for at least six times and repeat the forward grouping. Even then if the blood group discrepancy is not resolved, cell can be treated with DTT to remove the cold antibody (dithiothreitol, DTT breaks the IgM antibody).

PRACTICAL PROTOCOL FOR RESOLUTION OF BLOOD GROUP DISCREPANCY

Blood grouping and unknown irregular antibodies screening test of unknown serum (recipient/donor) through tube technique (CTT).

Procedure

- Prepare 2–5% of red blood cells suspension for forward grouping, Rh typing and autocontrol (prefer 5% of red blood cells suspension for serological tube testing).
- Prepare 5% of 'A_1', 'A_2' and 'B' blood group pooled red blood cells for reverse grouping and 'O' pooled red blood cells for unknown antibody and Bombay group screening (for donor and recipient).
- Take precipitin test tubes or standard glass test tubes and arrange serially from left-to-right direction according to the mark in a wooden rack.
- The wooden rack has been already marked 'A', 'B', AB', 'A_1', 'H', 'D_1' and 'D_2' (Rh) for cells grouping, 'A_1' cells, 'A_2' cells, 'B' cells, for serum grouping, 'O' cells, 'O' cells + Papain cysteine enzyme for antibody screening and Auto control (Donor/Recipient, self serum and self cell). Label the test tubes similarly.
- Mark sample number on all tubes by marker.
- Add prepared 2–5% of red blood cell suspension using clean pasture pipette or micropipette and place one drop (or 50 µl) of red cells for grouping, Rh typing and auto-control according to the labelled test tubes (prefer 5% of red blood cells suspension for serological tube testing).
- Collect unknown test serum (donor/recipient) using pasture pipette or micropipette and place two drops (or 100 µl) in serum grouping, antibody screening and auto-control in each tube.
- Prefer fresh samples for testing and do not use the hemolysed serum and hemolysed red blood cells suspension for blood centre serological tests.
- Take two drops (or 100 µl) of respected antisera 'A', 'B', 'AB', 'A_1', 'H', 'D_1' (IgM) and 'D_2' (Blend IgG + IgM) according to the labelled test tubes and in 5% of 'A_1' cells,

'A_2'cells, 'B' cells for reverse grouping and 'O' blood group pooled red blood cells for irregular unknown antibody (IgM) screening.

- Take one drop (or 50 µl) of papain cysteine enzyme before adding 'O' +ve pooled red blood cells suspension in serum tube for irregular unknown antibody (IgG) screening test.
- Take one drop (or 50 µl) 5% of red blood cell suspension (donor/recipient) in last serum tube for auto-control test and mix all the tubes gently.
- For Rh typing shake 'D' tube gently and centrifuge at 1000 rpm for one minute and read agglutination immediately macroscopically and microscopically and follow the manufacturer's instruction documented in the literature.
- Always use two different lots of same manufacturer or two different manufacturer's anti-'D' (monoclonal-IgM) and anti-D (blend IgG + IgM) for Rh (D) typing test which is mandatory according to drug control norm.
- 5% of pooled 'O' group red blood cells should be always used for the reverse grouping to rule out unknown antibodies and Bombay group (H).

NB: Spin method for cells and serum grouping—for cells grouping and serum grouping all the tubes are shaken gently and kept for minimum 15 minutes at room temperature as per model standard operating procedure for blood transfusion service guidelines and also follow the manufacturer's instruction. The test should be done at room temperature (20 to 24°C). And centrifuge at 1000 rpm for one minute and observe the agglutination.

Practical instruction

Forward grouping, reverse grouping + antibody screening + autocontrol (Figs 5.1, 5.2 and Table 5.2).

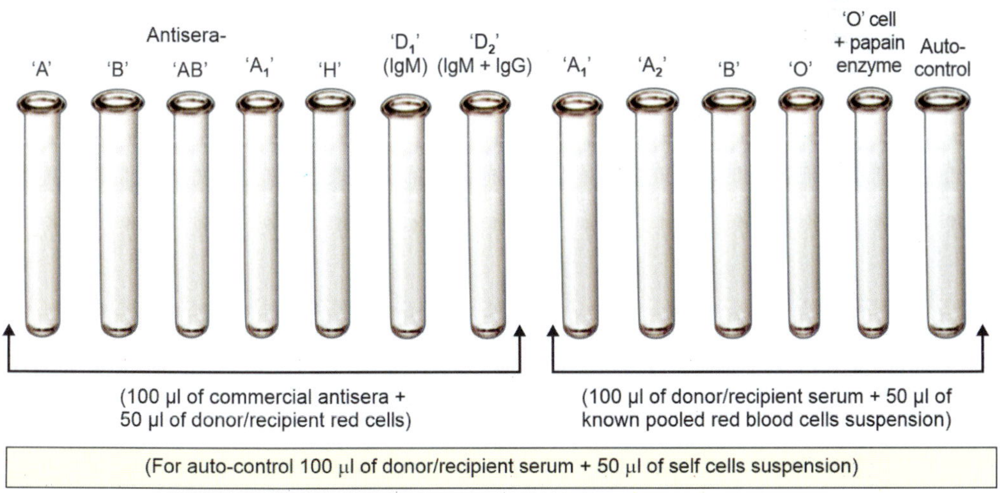

Fig. 5.1: Forward grouping, reverse grouping + antibody screening + autocontrol

BOMBAY GROUP

Discovered in 1952 in Mumbai by scientists Dr Bhende and Dr Bhatia.

There are always non-secretors of A, B, and H substances.

Table 5.2: Forward grouping, reverse grouping + antibody screening + autocontrol

Cell grouping (Antisera monoclonal)							*Serum/reverse grouping (Antibody screening, donor/recipient)*							
Anti 'A'	*Anti 'B'*	*Anti 'AB'*	*'A_1' lectin*	*'H' lectin*	*Anti 'D_1'(Rh) (IgM)*	*Anti 'D_2' (Rh) (IgM + IgG)*	*Group*	*'A_1' cell*	*'A_2' cell*	*'B' cell*	*'O' cell*	*'O' cell + Papain enzyme*	*Auto-control (self serum + self cell)*	*Group sustain*
+	–	+	+	+w	+	+	**A_1**	–	–	+	–	–	–	**'A_1' Rh +ve**
+	–	+	–	+	–	–	**A_2**	–	–	+	–	–	–	**'A_2' Rh –ve**
–	–	–	–	+	+	+	**O**	+	+	+	–	–	–	**'O' Rh +ve**
–	+	+	–	+w	+	+	**B**	+	+	–	–	–	–	**'B' Rh+ve**
+	+	+	+	+w	+	+	**A_1B**	–	–	–	–	–	–	**'A_1 B' Rh +ve**
+	+	+	–	+	+	+	**A_2B**	–	–	–	–	–	–	**'A_2 B' Rh +ve**
–	–	–	–	–	+	+	**Oh**	+	+	+	+	–	–	**'Oh' Rh +ve**

Note:

1. O cell with enzyme is not used routinely.
2. IAT of donor plasma/serum is tested with pooled O cell to detect presence of unexpected antibody and the result should be mentioned in the master record

It resembles 'O' blood group in the forward grouping but red blood cells additionally show a negative reaction when tested with anti-H lectin. But in reverse grouping agglutinates with 'O' red cells.

Anti 'H' antibody is always present in the plasma of the Bombay group person. 'H' antigen is missing. 'H' antigen is more visible agglutination in the case of 'O', 'A_2' and 'A_2 B' blood group, but 'A_1', 'A_1 B', and 'B' visible weaker agglutination.

'H' Ag strength O > A_2 > A_1 > A_2B > A_1B.

Other antisera like anti-AB, lectines anti-A_1 is used to resolve blood group discrepancy.

UNKNOWN IRREGULAR ANTIBODIES SCREENING TEST OF UNKNOWN SERUM (RECIPIENT/DONOR) BY STANDARD TUBE TECHNIQUE

Principle

The antibody screening test is used in the detection of unexpected antibodies. In this test, the donor's/patient's serum is tested using pooled 'O' red blood cells or the antibody-screening reagent red blood cells. The addition of a potentiating medium (enzyme/albumin) helps to promote the interaction of red blood cells and antibodies allowing antibody/antigen reactions to occur early. Positive reactions (hemolysis or agglutinations) in any tests indicate the presence of an all antibody or autoantibody in the serum.

1. Usually, two volumes of serum and one volume of 2–5% of red blood cells suspension in normal saline are used for optimum reaction (prefer 5% of red blood cells suspension for serological tube testing, whereas an equal volume of serum and 2–3% red cell suspension in LISS is used.
2. If antibodies screening cells shows positive in saline, enzyme, and IAT then further proceed for identification of atypical antibody detection through antibody identification panel cells.
3. Detection and identification of atypical antibodies. Possibility of antibodies present in serum.
   a. Incompatible cross-match
   b. Transfusion reaction
   c. Positive DAT result of the patient following transfusion
   d. Blood group discrepancy due to extra reaction with 'O' cell in reverse grouping
   e. History of multiple transfusion
   f. Pregnancy
   g. Identified alloantibody in the previous transfusion
   h. Rh incompatibility
4. System reacts through saline (IgM): M, N, P1, Le^a and Le^b,
   Enzyme (IgG): Rh system reacts like C, c, D, E, e.
   IAT (IgG): Ss, Kell, Kidd, Jk^a and Jk^b, Fy^a and Fy^b, Le^a and Le^b, and also reacts Rh system like C, c, D, E, e.

- Antibody screening (IgM) by 5% of 'O' blood group pooled red blood cells suspension + serum tubes are kept for 45 minutes at room temperature (22°C), centrifuge 1000 rpm post-incubation for one minute and observed for agglutination. It is used for detecting irregular unknown antibodies in the saline phase (IgM). Also, follow the instruction of the blood centre SOP.

- If serum + 'O' blood group pooled red blood cells suspension tubes show agglutination, then the Bombay group should be ruled out by testing for 'H' antigen with anti-H lectin.
- Used one special tube of 5% of 'O' pooled red blood cells suspension (+ papain cysteine enzyme if available) for detection of irregular unknown antibody (IgG).
- Take one drop (or 50 µl) of papain cysteine enzyme before adding 5% of 'O' +ve pooled red blood cells suspension in the serum tube and mix the tube gently.
- **Antibody screening (IgG):** Incubate the tube having serum + 5% of 'O' pooled red blood cells suspension + papain cysteine enzyme at 37°C for 45 minutes, centrifuge at 1000 rpm for one minute and observe the agglutination.
  - If agglutination is present, allo-antibody is suspected.
  - If the antibody specificity is in the Rh, Kidd, lewis blood group system, there is an enhanced reaction using the papain cysteine enzyme.
  - Certain red blood cell antigens including M, N, S, Xg^a and Fy^a and Fy^b are denatured (destroyed) when exposed to proteolytic enzymes.
- Antibody screening (IgG) serum +5% of 'O' pooled red blood cells suspension incubate at 37°C for one hour, centrifuge at 1000 rpm for one minute, and observe the agglutination.
  - If there is no agglutination, then it has to be taken ahead for IAT.
  - Wash the content thrice with normal saline and decant the supernatant completely and then add AHG.
  - Observe for agglutination. If agglutination is present, alloantibody is suspected.
  - **Temperature:** IgM antibodies react optimally at or below 22°C where as IgG reacts best at 37°C.
- **Use of autocontrol:** Autocontrol means incubation of the patients own cells and serum. Self-serum and self 2–5% wash red blood cells suspension is taken (prefer 5% of red blood cells suspension for serological tube testing).

Autocontrol is tested to rule out the presence of autoantibody detection and group discrepancies. Autocontrol is tested at three different temperatures, i.e. 4°C, 22°C, and 37°C to know the thermal activity of the autoantibody. If agglutination is detected at 37°C, it is a warm antibody. If agglutination is detected at 4°C, it is a cold antibody. The mixed antibody is reactive at both 4°C and 37°C (two drops of patient self-serum and one drop of self 5% red blood cells' suspension) in the precipitin tube, mixed well, incubate as per blood centre SOP and centrifuged at 1000 rpm for one minute and observe the agglutination.

Result

- If there is no agglutination, then autoantibody is absent.
- If agglutination is present then possibility of autoantibody is there and further DAT and IAT tests are done for the detection of incomplete antibody. If DAT strength (gradation of agglutination/clumps) is more than IAT, it is most suggestive of autoantibody.
- If IAT strength (gradation of agglutination/clumps) is more than DAT, alloantibody is suspected, for which antibody screening and identification is required.
- In the case of autoantibody, underlying alloantibody should be ruled out by autologous or allogenic adsorption test.

- Autocontrol is positive with serum consisting of antibodies against preservative (anti-LISS).

Figure 5.2 shows wooden rack with precipitin tubes or standard tubes.

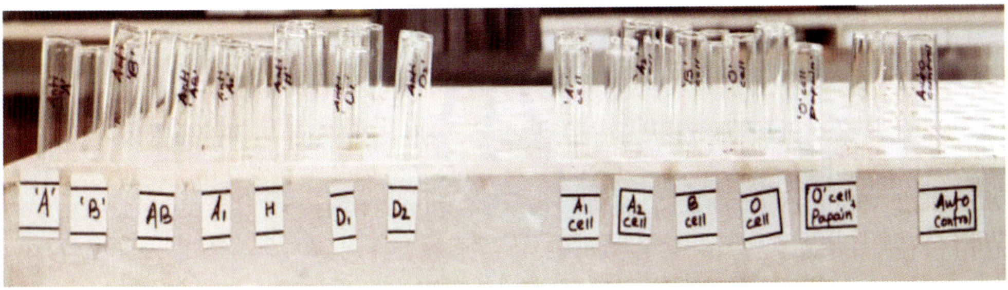

Fig. 5.2: Wooden rack with precipitin tubes or standard tubes

Chapter 6

Adsorption and Elution Test for Subgroup Analysis

ABO subgroups differ in the amount of antigen expression on red cells and, for secretors, soluble antigen present in the saliva.

Subgroups of A are more commonly encountered than subgroups of B.

The two principal subgroups of A are A_1 and A_2. Both these subgroups react with anti-A strongly whereas the A_1 subgroup is differentiated from A_2 by testing with anti-A_1 lectin. Subgroups other than A_2 occur infrequently.

Generally, the classification of weak A subgroups (A_3, Ax, Am, Ael) is based on the:

1. The amount of A antigen present on red cells which is reflected by
   - The degree of red cell agglutination by anti-A and anti-A_1.
   - The degree of red cell agglutination by human and some monoclonal anti-A, B.
2. The amount of H antigen present on red cells which is reflected by the degree of red cell agglutination by anti-H (*Ulex europaeus*).
3. Presence or absence of anti-A_1 in the serum.
4. Presence of A and H substances in the saliva of secretors.
5. Adsorption/elution studies.
6. Family (pedigree) studies.

Adsorption/Elution Studies

Principle: ABO subgroups are the phenotypes with weak expression of antigens that cannot be detected by conventional serological test, or even after incubating in cold temperature or increase with cell concentration. The presence of A or B antigens, can be detected by adsorbing them with anti-A or anti-B to red blood cells, followed by elution of the bound antibody. The eluate is then evaluated for the presence of ant-A and anti-B by testing with A or B pooled red blood cells.

Reagents/Apparatus Required

- Pilot test tubes and precipitin test tubes or standard test tubes.
- Wooden rack and test tube rack.
- Micropipette and pasture pipette.
- Digital table-top centrifuge machine.

- Digital display incubator.
- Digital temperature control water bath (56°C).
- 5% of 'A', 'B', and 'O' blood group pooled red blood cell suspension.
- Anti- 'A', and Anti-'B'/polyclonal (human serum).
- 2–3 pooled 'A' and 'B' blood group serum.
- 0.9% chilled normal saline.

Adsorption Technique

Step 1

- Wash the patient's red blood cells 3–4 times with normal saline and discard the supernatant fluid.
- Take an equal volume of 8–10 drops (or 500 µl) of the patient's packed red blood cell and 8–10 drops (or 500 µl) of polyclonal antiserum using a clean standard pasture pipette or micropipette in tube. The pooled serum used is against the corresponding antigen to be detected.
- Suppose, the forward grouping shows weaker/no agglutination with antisera A, but the reverse grouping (reaction with 'B' blood group red cells) suggestive of 'A' blood group then use pooled serum of 'B' blood group (polyclonal anti-'A') for adsorption test.
- Similarly, suppose the forward grouping shows weaker/no agglutination with antisera B, but the reverse grouping (reaction with 'A' blood group red cells). Suggestive of 'B', blood group then use pooled serum of 'A' blood group for adsorption test. Mix well gently.
- Incubate at 4°C temperature for one hour.

Step 2

Preparation of adsorbed cells:

- Centrifuge the patient's packed red blood cells mixed with the required group of pooled serum tubes at 3,000–4,000 RPM for 5 minutes.
- Immediately separate the serum in the supernatant by micropipette or clean pasture pipette and keep it in a separate precipitin tube or standard test tube.
- After removing the serum wash the (antibody-coated) packed red blood cells with chilled saline. (Keep saline in blood centre freeze at 4°C minimum 4–6 hours before the test run.)
- Wash the antibody-coated red blood cells 3–4 times in a large volume of chilled saline at 3,000–4,000 RPM for 3–4 minutes and collect the last supernatant (chilled saline) from the tube as much as possible and keep in separate tube.

Preparation of supernatant from last wash:

- The last wash (supernatant) should be checked by known 'A' or 'B' pooled red blood cells and the result should be negative. If any reaction is there further washing is needed. (This last wash is an important negative control that demonstrates that the residual unbound antibody has been removed and it will not interfere with the elute that is to be prepared from the washed red blood cells.)

Step 3

Elution technique

Materials:

- 6% of bovine albumin prepared by diluting from 22% of bovine albumin with saline (1.4 ml 22% bovine albumin + 3.6 ml normal saline) or pooled 'AB' group serum.
- Test tube
- Serological water bath
- Supernatant from the last wash is kept to test the validity of elution.

Methodology

Prepare warm saline:

- Switch on the water bath and adjust the temperature to 56°C.
- When the temperature becomes 56°C in the water bath, keep the saline bottle in a water bath for 5–10 minutes.
- In the tube containing washed packed red cells, add an equal volume of normal saline or neutral 'AB' blood group serum or 6% of bovine albumin using a clean pasture pipette or micropipette (6% of bovine albumin is preferred for elute preparation). Then warm saline or 'AB' blood group serum or 6% bovine albumin is added to the tube, and placed in the water-bath at 56°C for 5–10 minutes with frequent mixing.
- If elute is used the same day, it can be prepared in saline, if storage is anticipated elute is prepared in AB serum or in 6% of bovine albumin.
- After completion of incubation, centrifuge immediately at 3,000–4,000 rpm (try putting RCF values as rpms change from centrifuge-to-centrifuge) for 2–3 minutes.
- Immediately transfer the supernatant elute fluid by clean pasture pipette or autopipette in a precipitin test tube (supernatant looks like hemolysed one).
- Take three precipitin test tubes and mark then as 'A', 'B', and 'O'.
- Add one drop (or 50 µl) of prepared elute (haemolysed supernatant) according to these tubes.
- Add one drop (or 50 µl) of prepared 5% of 'A', 'B', and 'O' pooled red blood cell suspension according to the mark in tubes.
- Mix gently.
- 'O' pooled red blood cells are used for control.
- Incubate at room temperature for 20–30 minutes.
- Centrifuge at 1000 rpm for one minute and observe the result.

Interpretation

If the patient is a suspected case of A^{weaker} blood group and adsorption elution test also found a weaker variant of 'A' then reporting is Aw blood group (Table 6.1).

Table 6.1: Example of weaker variant test result

Weak reaction of antigen	*Antisera used*	*Reaction of eluate with*	*Interpretation*
A	Anti-A	A cell	A/AB subgroup
B	Anti-B	B cell	B subgroup

Note: A_1 is the commonest subgroup (80%) followed by A_2 (20%) and the other weaker A subgroups are A_3, Ax, Am, Ael.

Chapter 7

Titration Technique of ABO and Rh Antibodies

Basic Principle of Antibody Titration Technique

Titration is a semi-quantitative method used to determine the concentration of antibodies in a serum sample or to compare the strength of antigen expression on different red cell samples.

Utility of Titration and Technique of Steps in Blood Centre Serology

The titration technique is an important methodology for blood centre serology, immunohematology, and microbiology. In blood centre serology, titration is required to detect the strength of antibodies like anti-'A', anti-'B', anti-'H' and Rh antibodies (anti-D, and quality control of blood grouping antisera, and also in preparation and standardization of lectin *Dolichos biflorus* (A1 lectin). Antibody titration is also performed to monitor hemolytic disease of newborn (Rh HDN, ABO HDN). The tube technique for titration is the best and most reliable technique.

TECHNIQUES OF ANTIBODIES AND ANTISERA TITRATION

- Take 11 precipitin test tubes or standard glass test tubes as per the requirement and label them as 1-in 2-to 1-in-1024. Leaving the 1st tube as 1 in 1 (labelled as neat) in this row.
- For proper titration reaction, two drops (or 100 µl) normal saline in all tubes leaving the 1st tube (labelled as neat) in this row, add two drops of serum/antisera in 1st and 2nd tubes (dilution 1-in-1 and 1-in-2), mix well transfer two drops (or 100 µl) of diluted serum/antisera from 2nd tube (labelled as 1 in 2) to 3rd tube.
- Repeat this same process up to 11th tube.
- Take two drops (or 100 µl) from 11th tube and discard it or save for further dilution if required.
- Add one drop (or 50 µl) of prepared 2–5% of corresponding red blood cells suspension in all tubes from neat to remaining tubes (prefer 5% of red blood cells suspension for serological tube testing).
- Incubate at room temperature (for anti-A and anti-B titers) or 37°C (for IgG titer) for 45 minutes.
- Centrifuge all the test tubes with 1000 rpm for one minute.
- Observe the macroscopic agglutination, the last test tube showing visible agglutination, marked as the titration of the sample.

- For AHG method to detect IgG Abs, wash the tubes with saline after incubation and add 2 drops (or 100 µl) of AHG. Centrifuge and read the agglutination.
- The titration results should be read from lesser concentration to higher concentration.

Steps of Titration

Titration of known A, B, and O blood group antibodies in saline preparation (IgM).

The master dilution/serial dilution technique for titration studies is as follows:

- Careful pipetting is essential. Pipettes with disposable tips that can be changed after each dilution are recommended.
- Optimal temperature and duration of incubation, and force and duration of centrifugation must be used consistently.
- Label 10 test tubes according to the serum dilution (e.g. 1-in-1, 1-in-2, etc).
- A 1-in-1 dilution means one volume of serum undiluted; a 1-in-2 dilution means one volume of serum in a final volume of two.
- Deliver one volume of saline to all test tubes except the first (undiluted 1-in-1) tube.
- Add an equal volume of serum to the first two tubes (undiluted and 1-in-2).
- Using a clean pipette, mix the contents of the 1-in-2 dilution several times and transfer one volume into the next tube (the 1-in-4 dilutions).
- Continue the same process for all dilutions, using a clean pipette to mix and transfer each dilution. Remove one volume of diluted serum from the final tube and save it for use if further dilutions are required.
- Label 10 tubes for the appropriate dilutions.
- Using separate pipettes for each dilution, transfer 2 drops of each diluted serum into the appropriately labelled tubes and add one drop of a 5% red cell suspension. Mix well and centrifuge at 1000 rpm for 1 min. Observe the agglutination and the tube showing the least macroscopic (naked eye) agglutination is depicted as the titer of that antibody.

Note: 2–5% of corresponding Rh-positive pooled red blood cells suspension is used for 'A', 'B', 'O' and Bombay group antibodies titer. Red cells that express the antigen(s) corresponding to the antibody specificity(ies), in a 2 to 5% saline suspension. Uniformity of cell suspensions is very important to ensure comparability of results.

Example of red cell suspension used for antibody titer: For 'A' blood group antibodies titer 'B' blood group pooled red blood cells is used, 'B' blood group antibodies titer 'A' blood group pooled red cells is used, 'O' blood group antibodies titer 'A' and 'B' blood group pooled red cells are used, Bombay group antibodies titer 'A', 'B' and 'O' group pooled red cells are used. There is an antigen on both the sides ('A' and 'B' sides) of 'AB' blood group but no antibody, so it does not need any antibody titer.

For 'A' Blood Group Antibodies

Reagents/Apparatus required

1. 2 pilot tubes (12 × 100 mm) and 11 precipitin tubes or standard glass tubes.
2. Wooden rack and test tube rack.
3. Micropipette or pasture pipette.

4. Digital bench top centrifuge machine.
5. 2–5% of corresponding Rh-positive pooled red blood cell suspension.
6. Known 'A' blood group serum.
7. 0.9% normal saline.
   - Take 11 precipitin test tubes or standard glass test tubes and arrange them serially in a vertical position from the left-to-right direction in a horizontal wooden rack.
   - Mark on the test tubes from 1st to 11th by marker. 1st test tube labelled as neat (Fig. 7.1).
   - Deliver two drops (or 100 µl) of normal saline (0.9%) using a standard pasture pipette or using micropipette from 2nd (labelled as 1-in-2) to 11th test tubes leaving the 1st test tube in this row, labelled as 1-in-2 to 1-in-1024.
   - Add two drops (or 100 µl) of known 'A' blood group serum by standard pasture pipettes or using micropipette in 1st and 2nd tubes.
   - Do not use the haemolysed serum.
   - Mix gently serum with saline in 2nd test tube without bubble formation.
   - Take two drops (or 100 µl) of diluted serum from 2nd tube and transfer into 3rd tube. Repeat this same process up to 11th tube. Take two drops (or 100 µl) from the 11th tube and discard it or save it for further dilution if required.
   - For anti 'B' antibody titration in a 'A' blood group individual use 2–5% of corresponding known 'B' blood group pooled red blood cells suspension and add one drop (or 50 µl) to all tubes from 1st to 11th and mix gently all thoroughly (prefer 5% of red blood cells suspension for serological tube testing).
   - Do not use the hemolysed cell suspension.
   - Keep the tubes in room temperature (20–24°C) for 45 minutes, centrifuge at 1000 rpm for one minute, and observe the result macroscopically and microscopically. Follow the manufacturer's instructions documented in the literature.
   - Similarly, apply for 'B' blood group antibodies titer anti 'A' titration use 2–5% of 'A' blood group pooled red blood cells suspension. For 'O' blood group antibodies titer use 2–5% of 'A' and 'B' blood group pooled red blood cells suspension and the process requires 22 tubes, for Bombay group antibodies titer use 2–5% of 'A', 'B', and 'O' blood group pooled red blood cells suspension and it requires 33 test tubes (prefer 5% of red blood cells suspension for serological tube testing).
   - Follow the above-mentioned instructions and steps for 'B', 'O' and Bombay group (H) antibodies.

Practical Instruction for 'A' Blood Group Antibodies

- 1st tube 1-in-1 which has only serum and cell suspension is called neat.
- From 2nd tube to 11th tubes according to serial number left-to-right direction titer is 1-in-2, 1-in-4, 1-in-8, 1-in-16, 1-in-32, 1-in-64, 1-in-128, 1-in-256, 1-in-512, 1-in-1024, respectively.
- Follow the above-mentioned instructions or steps for 'O', 'B' and Bombay group (H) antibodies.

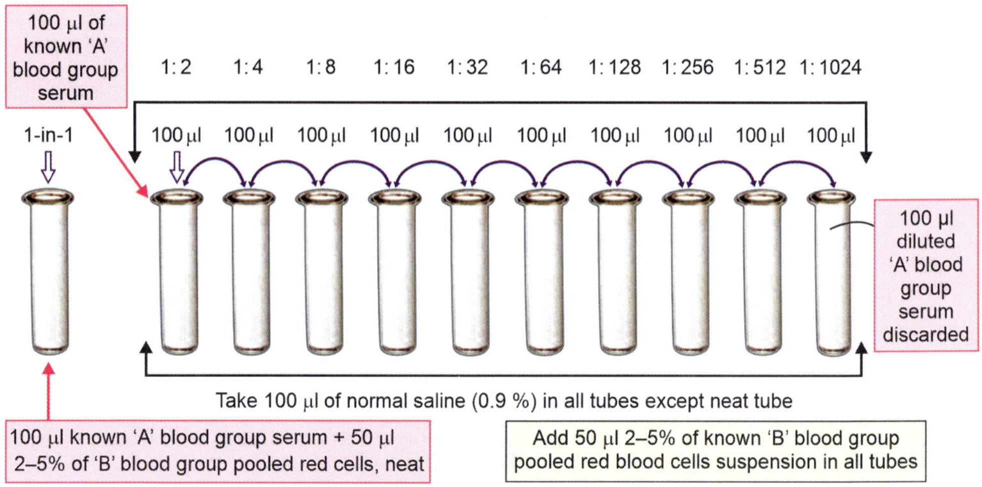

Fig. 7.1: Practical instruction for 'A' blood group antibodies

Interpretation of titration result:

- Observe the highest dilution that produces macroscopic agglutination.
- The titer is reciprocal of the dilution level, e.g. 32 for 1-in-32.
- If there is agglutination in the tube containing the most diluted serum, the end-point has not been reached, and the additional dilution should be prepared and tested.

Uses of Low Titer Type 'O' Whole Blood

1. Anti-A and anti-B antibodies are tested in the laboratory for each donation to determine whether the individual blood product contains a low titer of ABO antibodies.

   Low titer type 'O' group whole blood means the complete product contains type 'O' red blood cells and plasma containing low levels of antibodies making it safe to transfuse to a patient with any blood type. There are anti-A and anti-B antibodies present in the plasma of type 'O' group donors. In low titer type 'O' whole blood products, the antibodies are tested to be at low, safe levels.

   This product has proven advantages to save lives in emergency trauma cases.
2. Low titer type 'O' group whole blood is most commonly used in trauma cases where massive blood loss has occurred, such as in hospital emergency rooms.
3. If a donor's isoagglutinin titer is high, then avoid issuing whole blood or plasma or platelet to a patient of minor mismatch .

Example: If the recipient's blood group is 'A' or 'B' or 'AB' and the donor unit is 'O' blood group, it is a minor mismatch transfusion. ABO antibody titer levels more than 64 is considered high titer and called dangerous O group.

Titration of Rh Antibodies in Saline Preparation (IgM)

Reagents/Apparatus required

1. Two pilot test tubes (12 × 100 mm) and 11 precipitin test tubes or standard glass test tubes.
2. Wooden rack and test tube rack.

3. Micropipette or pasture pipette.
4. Digital table top centrifuge machine.
5. Digital display incubator.
6. 2–5% of corresponding 'O' blood group Rh-positive pooled red blood cells suspension.
7. Unknown test serum.
8. 0.9% normal saline.

- Take 11 precipitin test tubes or standard glass test tubes and arrange them serially in vertical position from left-to-right direction in horizontal wooden rack.
- Mark on the test tubes 1st to11th by the marker. 1st test tube was labelled as neat (Fig. 7.2).
- Deliver two drops (or 100 µl) of normal saline (0.9%) using a standard pasture pipette or using micropipette from 2nd (labelled as 1-in-2) to 11th tubes leaving the 1st tube in this row, labelled as 1-in-2 to 1-in-1024.
- Add two drops (or 100 µl) of unknown test serum using a standard pasture pipette or using micropipette in 1st and 2nd test tubes.
- Do not use the hemolysed serum.
- Mix gently serum with saline in 2nd tube.
- Take two drops (or 100 µl) of diluted sample from the 2nd tube and transfer into 3rd test tube. Repeat this same process up to 11th test tube.
- Take two drops (or 100 µl) from the 11th tube and discard it or save for further dilution if required.
- Add one drop (or 50 µl) of 2–5% of 'O' blood group Rh-positive pooled red blood cells suspension in all tubes from 1st to 11th (prefer 5% of red blood cells suspension for serological tube testing).
- Mix gently all tubes and incubate at 37°C for 45 minutes.
- And also follow the instruction of the blood centre SOP.

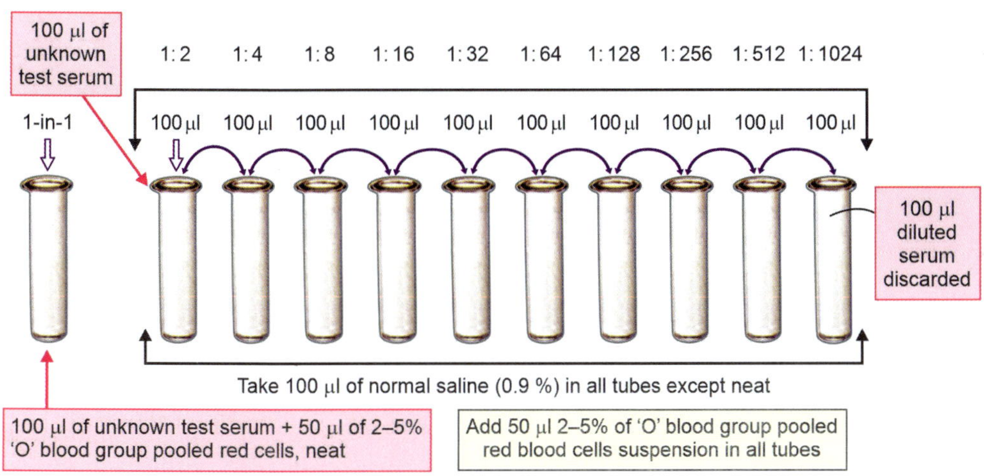

Fig. 7.2: Titration of Rh antibodies in saline preparation

- Do not use the hemolysed cells suspension.
- After incubation centrifuge at 1000 rpm for one minute and observe the result macroscopically and microscopically.

Practical Instruction of Rh Antibodies in Saline Preparation

- 1st test tube which has only serum and red blood cells suspension is called neat. From 2nd to 11th tubes according to serial number left-to-right direction titer is 1-in-2, 1- in-4, 1-in-8, 1-in-16, 1-in-32, 1-in-64, 1-in-128, 1-in-256, 1-in-512, 1-in-1024, respectively.

Titration of Rh Antibodies in Papain Cystin Enzyme Preparation (IgG)

Follow the above mentioned saline antibodies reagent and apparatus and extra papain cysteine enzyme reagent needed in enzyme preparation.

- Take 11 precipitin test tubes or standard glass tubes and arrange serially on vertical position from left to the right direction in a horizontal wooden rack.
- Mark on the tubes 1st to 11th by marker. 1st tube is labelled as neat (Fig. 7.3).
- Deliver two drops (or 100 µl) of normal saline (0.9%) using a standard pasture pipette or using micropipette from 2nd (labelled as 1-in-2) to 11th tubes leaving the 1st tube in this row, labelled as 1-in-2 to 1-in-1024.
- Add two drops (or 100 µl) of unknown test serum using a standard pasture pipette or using micropipette in 1st and 2nd tubes.
- Dc not use the hemolysed serum.
- Mix gently normal saline and test serum in the second tube.
- From 2nd tube take two drops (or 100 µl) of diluted sample and transfer in to third tube. This process is done up to 11th tube. From 11th tube two drops (or 100 µl) discard it or save for further dilution if required.
- Add one drop (or 50 µl) of papain cysteine enzyme in each tube from 1st to 11th.
- Add one drop (or 50 µl) 2–5% of 'O' blood group Rh-positive pooled red blood cells suspension in all tubes from 1st to 11th tubes (prefer 5% of red blood cells suspension for serological tube testing).
- Do not use the hemolysed cell suspension.
- Mix gently all tubes and incubate at 37°C for 45 minutes.
- After incubation centrifuge at 1000 rpm for one minute and read the titer result macroscopically and microscopically.

Practical instruction of Rh antibodies in papain cysteine enzyme preparation

1st test tube which has only serum and red blood cells suspension is called neat. From 2nd to 11th tubes according to serial number left to right direction, titer is 1-in-2, 1-in-4, 1-in-8, 1-in-16, 1-in-32, 1-in-64, 1-in-128, 1-in-256, 1-in-512, 1-in-1024, respectively.

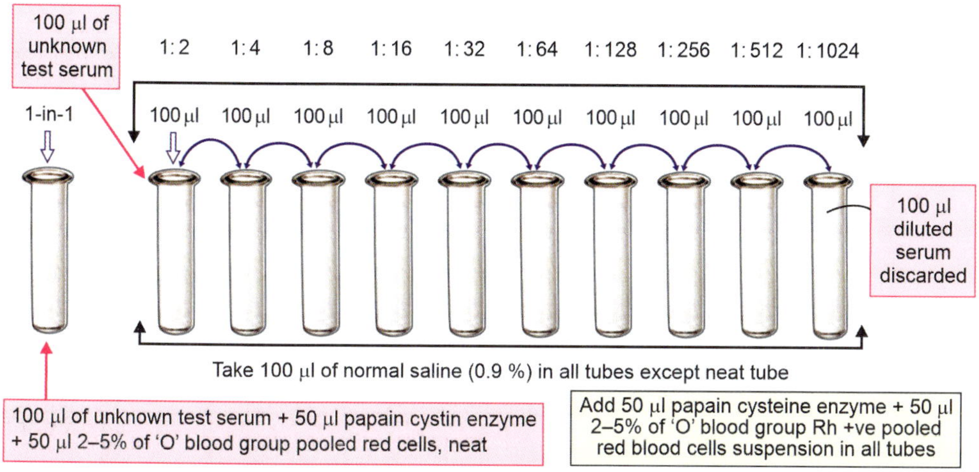

Fig. 7.3: Practical instruction of Rh antibodies in papain cysteine enzyme

Titration of Anti-D by Indirect Antiglobulin Test (IgG)

Follow the above-mentioned saline antibodies reagent and apparatus, extra AHG reagent and 5% of 'O' blood group Rh +ve pooled red blood cells suspension needed in IAT preparation.

- Take 11 precipitin test tubes or standard glass tubes and arrange them serially in a vertical position from left-to-right direction in a horizontal wooden rack.
- Mark on the tubes 1st to 11th by marker. 1st tube was labelled as neat.
- Deliver two drops (or 100 µl) of normal saline (0.9%) using standard pasture pipette using micropipette from 2nd (labelled as 1-in-2) to 11th tubes leaving the 1st tube in this row, labelled as 1-in-2 to 1-in-1024.
- Add two drops (or 100 µl) of unknown test serum using a standard pasture pipette or using micropipette in 1st and 2nd tubes.
- Mix gently serum with saline in 2nd tube.
- Do not use the haemolysed serum.
- Take two drops (or 100 µl) of diluted sample from 2nd tube and transfer in to 3rd tube. Repeat this same process up to 11th tube. Take two drops (or 100 µl) from 11th tube and discard it or save for further dilution if required.
- Add one drop (or 50 µl) 5% of 'O' blood group Rh-positive pooled red blood cells suspension in all tubes from 1st to 11th tubes.
- Do not use the haemolysed cells suspension.
- Mix gently all the tubes and incubate at 37°C for 1 hour.
- After incubation washes the red blood cells 3–4 times in a large volume of normal saline.
- Decant the supernatant fluid from tubes as much as possible.
- After last wash add two drops or (100 µl) of anti-human globulin (AHG) in all tubes including neat tube to the red cells button.
- Centrifuge at 1000 rpm for one minute all the tubes and observe the agglutination macroscopically and microscopically.
- Keep +ve and –ve controls for Rh antibodies.

+ Ve control

Take precipitin tube or standard tube

100 µl of anti D (IgG) monoclonal

+

50 µl of 5% O +
blood group pooled red cells

↓

Incubate 37°C for 1 hour

↓

Wash 3–4 times

↓

Add 100 µl of AHG

↓

Centrifuge 1000 rpm for 1 minute

↓

Observe the agglutination
(agglutination should be seen)

- Ve control

Take precipitin tube or standard tube

100 µl of 6% bovine albumin

+

50 µl of 5% O –
blood group pooled red cells

↓

Incubate 37°C for 1 hour

↓

Wash 3–4 times

↓

Add 100 µl of AHG

↓

Centrifuge 1000 rpm for 1 minute

↓

Observe the agglutination
(No-Agglutination should be seen)

PRACTICAL INSTRUCTION

Anti-D (IgG Antibodies of pregnant mother) titer.

1st Step

- 1st test tube which has only serum and red blood cell suspension is called neat (Fig. 7.4). From 2nd tube to 11th tube according to serial number left to right direction titer is 1-in-2, 1-in-4, 1-in-8, 1-in-16, 1-in-32, 1-in-64, 1-in-128, 1-in-256, 1-in-512, 1-in-1024, respectively.

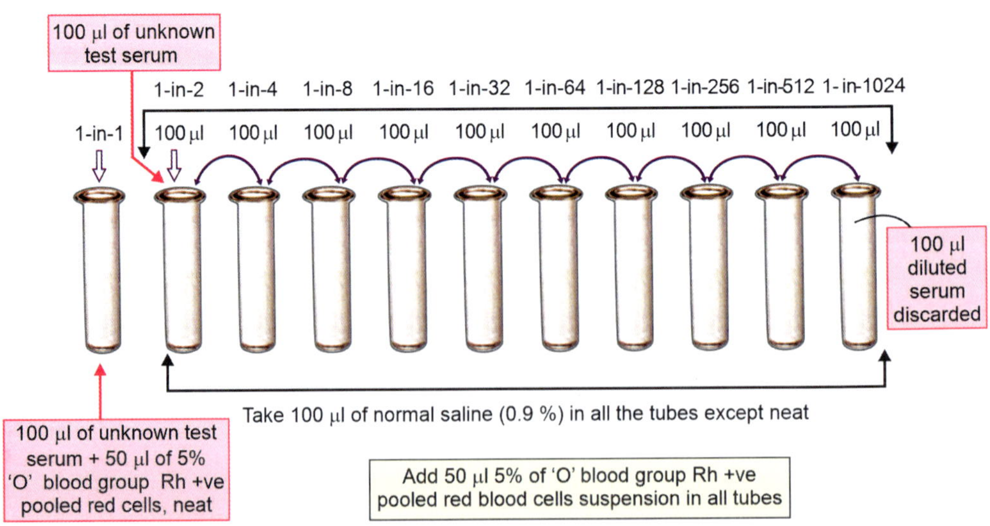

Fig. 7.4: Anti-D (IgG antibodies of pregnant mother) titer

- Incubate all tubes including neat at 37°C for 1 hour.
- After incubation wash all tubes 3–4 times with normal saline.

2nd Step

After last wash, add 100 µl of antihuman globulin (AHG) in all the tubes including neat.

- Centrifuge at 1000 rpm for one minute all the tubes and observe the agglutination macroscopically and microscopically.
- Keep +ve and –ve controls for Rh antibodies.
- Rh antibody titer is required for cases of:
  - Rh HDN (hemolytic disease of new-born baby):
    - If newborn baby's DAT is positive.
    - If the mother's serum antibody screening using 'O' red blood cells + serum and 'O' red blood cells + serum + papain cysteine enzyme shows positive agglutination.
    - If the mother has Rh –ve and the baby has Rh +ve.

Immunohematological Work-up for Rh HDN

- Cells grouping and serum grouping of the mother's sample.
- Cells grouping and DAT from cord sample. (Sample should be washed for 3–4 times with normal saline).
- Rh antibody titer of mother's serum by saline, enzyme and IAT method with positive and negative control.

Pathophysiology of Rh HDN

- When the mother is Rh-negative, baby is Rh-positive and the father is Rh-positive.

The baby got 'D' antigen on red blood cells from the father.

↓

The mother produces anti 'D' antibody. The first baby is unaffected.

- In subsequent pregnancy with Rh-D-positive baby, the IgG type antibody transferred through placenta and coats the RBC of the foetus.

↓

Destruction of red blood cells

↓

Anemia, jaundice

↓

Hemolytic disease of the fetus and newborn

Chapter 8

Secretor Status Studies Through Saliva Testing for A, B and H Substances

Inhibition Technique

Purpose: Whether patient is a secretor or non-secretor.

Principle: Secretor status can be determined through genotyping or through serological method, the person's saliva is boiled, then added to reagents containing antibodies against the A, B and H antigens. Red blood cells expressing these antigens are then added to the saliva-reagent mixtures. These secretor status of a person can be useful to determine certain doubtful cases of ABO blood grouping and also has clinical significant. The secretor status of an individual is also helpful to identify weaker varients of ABO grouping.

Reagents/Apparatus Required

1. Pilot test tubes, precipitin test tubes or standard glass test tubes.
2. Small beaker or wide-mouth 15 ml test tube and conical funnel.
3. Horizontal wooden rack and test tube rack.
4. Micropipette or pasture pipette.
5. Digital table top centrifuge machine.
6. Digital temperature control water bath (100°C).
7. 0.9% normal saline.
8. Antisera 'A', and 'B' human polyclonal and lectin 'H'.
9. 2–5% of 'A' , 'B', and 'O' pooled red blood cells suspension.

Step 1

Saliva collection technique:

- Before collecting saliva, ask the patient or donor to wash his/her mouth properly with clean water.
- A few grains of salt may be sprinkled on the tongue to induce salivation or ask to chew rubber.
- Advise to keep mouth shut for 5–10 minutes.
- Collect 5–10 ml of saliva in a wide-mouth test tube through clean sterile conical funnel or small beaker and put cover.
- Keep test tube or beaker containing saliva in a boiling water bath and boil at 100°C for 10 minutes to inactivate any enzymes present.

- Centrifuge the boiled saliva at 3000 rpm or 4000 rpm for 10 minutes.
- Collect clean supernatant through pasture pipette and transfer in separate test tube for further test procedure.

Step II

Titration

- Antisera 'A' titer with corresponding 2–5% of 'A' pooled red blood cells.
- Antisera 'B' titer with corresponding 2–5% of 'B' pooled red blood cells.
- Lectin 'H' titer with corresponding 2–5% of 'O' pooled red blood cells.

  (Prefer 5% of pooled red blood cells suspension for secretor studies).
- Titration steps should be followed as mentioned in Chapter 7.

Techniques of Antibodies and Antisera Titration

- Take 11 precipitin test tubes or standard glass test tubes as per the requirement and label them as 1-in-2 to 1-in-1024. Leaving the 1st tube as 1-in-1 (labelled as neat) in this row.
- For proper titration reaction, two drops (or 100 µl) normal saline in all tubes leaving the 1st tube (labelled as neat) in this row, two parts antisera add in 1st and 2nd tube (dilution 1 in 1 and 1-in-2), mix well transfer two drops (or 100 µl) of diluted antisera from 2nd tube (labelled as 1-in-2) and transfer in to 3rd tube.
- Repeat this same process up to 11th tube.
- Take two drops (or 100 µl) from 11th tube and discard it or save for further dilution if required.
- Add one part one drop (or 50 µl) of prepared 2–5% of corresponding red blood cells suspension in all tubes from neat to remaining tubes (prefer 5% of red blood cells suspension for serological tube testing).
- Add 5% pooled 'A' red blood cells suspension to all the tubes of antisera 'A'.
- Add 5% pooled 'B' red blood cells suspension to all the tubes of antisera 'B'.
- Add 5% pooled 'O' red blood cells suspension to all the tubes of lectin 'H'.
- Incubate at room temperature for 45 minutes.
- Centrifuge all the test tubes with 1000 rpm for one minute.
- **Read result:** Observe the macroscopic agglutination, the last test tube showing visible agglutination, marked as the titration of the sample.

  (The titration results should be read from lesser concentration to higher concentration.)

Step III

- Do titration of antisera 'A', antisera 'B' and lectin 'H'.
- Choose dilutions, where the strength of agglutination is 2+.
- This dilution of antisera is required for secretor status studies.

Formula:

Observe titre/required titer.

Saliva Dilution

Saliva from adult patients should be diluted 1-in-2, because undiluted saliva contains non-specific glycoproteins which may cause erroneous results.

Dilution technique of antisera with example:

If antisera 'A' observed titer 1-in-32 and require titer 1-in-8. $\frac{\cancel{32}\ 4}{\cancel{8}\ 1}$ = 1-in-4

In a serological test tube take 3 drops normal saline and 1 drop antisera 'A'.

Similarly, if antisera 'B' observed titer 1-in-64 and require titer 1-in-8. $\frac{\cancel{64}\ 8}{\cancel{8}\ 1}$ = 1-in-8

In a serological test tube take 7 drops normal saline and 1 drop antisera 'B'.

Similarly, if lectin 'H' observed titer 1-in-64 and require titer 1-in-8. $\frac{\cancel{64}\ 8}{\cancel{8}\ 1}$ = 1-in-8

In a serological test tube take 7 drops of normal saline and 1 drop of lectin 'H'.

Step IV

Method:

- Take 6 precipitin test tubes or standard serological glass test tubes and mark as test 'A', 'B' and 'H', and as control 'C_1', 'C_2' and 'C_3' (C = control tubes).
- In the 'A' test tube take 2 drops (or 100 µl) of diluted antisera 'A', in a 'B' test tube take 2 drops (or 100 µl) of diluted antisera 'B', in a 'H' test tube take 2 drops (or 100 µl) of diluted antisera 'H'
- Add 2 drops (or 100 µl) of saliva in all the three test tubes (A, B and H tubes).
- In the control tubes instead of saliva take normal saline.
- In 'C_1', C_2 and C_3 test tubes take 2 drops (or 100 µl) of normal saline and 2 drops (or 100 µl) of diluted antisera 'A' in C_1 test tube, 2 drops (or 100 µl) of diluted antisera 'B' in C_2 test tube and 2 drops (or 100 µl) of diluted lectin 'H' in C_3 test tube. Mix well all the tubes test and control and incubate at room temperature for 30 minutes.
- After incubation add 1 drop (or 50 µl) of 5% 'A' blood group pooled red blood cells suspension in 'A' and C_1 test tubes.
- Add 1 drop (or 50 µl) of 5% 'B' blood group pooled red blood cells suspension in 'B' and C_2 test tubes.
- Add 1 drop (or 50 µl) of 5% 'O' blood group pooled red blood cells suspension in 'H' and C_3 test tubes.
- Mix well all the tubes and again incubate in room temperature for one hour. Centrifuge at 1000 rpm for one minute and read result with macroscopically.

Interpretation

1. No agglutination in the test sample and agglutination in the corresponding control tubes indicates that the antiserum has been neutralized by the blood group specific substance A, B or H and the individual is secretor.

2. Agglutination in all the test sample and control tubes indicates that the absence of blood group substances and the person is nonsecretor or Bombay phenotype (Oh).

Example with explanation:

1. **'A' and 'H' test tubes show no-agglutination, but 'B' test tube shows agglutination and also control C_1, C_2 and C_3 test tubes show agglutination Result:** 'A' secretor.
2. **'B' and 'H' test tubes show no-agglutination, but 'A' test tube shows agglutination and also control C_1, C_2 and C_3 test tubes show agglutination. Result:** 'B' secretor.
3. **'A', 'B' and 'H' test tubes show no-agglutination and control C_1, C_2 and C_3 test tubes show agglutination. Result:** 'AB' secretor.
4. **'A' and 'B' test tubes show agglutination, but 'H' test tube shows no-agglutination and also control C_1, C_2 and C_3 test tubes show agglutination Result:** 'O' secretor.
5. **'A', 'B' and 'H' test tubes show agglutination and also control C_1, C_2 and C_3 test tubes show agglutination. Result:** Oh' nonsecretor (Bombay phenotype).

This example indicates the presence of A and H substances in the saliva and the individual is of blood group A. Similarly, B group secretor will secrete B and H substances and O group secretor will only have H substance in the saliva.

Chapter 9

Preparation of Sensitized Red Cells, IgG (Coombs Control Cell)

Principle

It is used for validity check of the DAT, IAT, and quality control checking of the AHG test. If DAT/IAT test result is negative, then the result is validated using this cell.

Reagents and Materials Required

1. Precipitin test tubes or standard glass test tubes.
2. Micropipette or pasture pipette.
3. Digital table top centrifuge machine.
4. Digital temperature control incubator.
5. Anti 'D' IgG monoclonal (can use only IgG anti 'D' for sensitization: IgM will agglutinate it so cannot use blend (IgG + IgM).
6. 3–5% 'O' Rh (D) positive pooled red blood cells.
7. Antihuman globulin (AHG).
8. 0.9% normal saline.

Preparation of Sensitized Red Cells

Step I

- Take 11 precipitin test tubes or standard glass test tubes and arrange them serially in a vertical position from the left-to-right direction in a horizontal wooden rack.
- Mark on the tubes 1st to 11th by marker. 1st tube is labelled as neat.
- Deliver two drops (or 100 µl) of normal saline (0.9%), using standard clean pasture pipette or using micropipette from 2nd (labelled as 1 in 2) to 11th tubes leaving the 1st tube in this row, labelled as 1-in-2 to 1 in 1024.
- Add two drops (or 100 µl) of antisera 'D' (IgG, monoclonal) using standard pasture pipette or using micropipette in 1st and 2nd tube.
- Mix gently antisera with normal saline in 2nd tube.
- Take two drops (or 100 µl) of diluted sample from 2nd tube and transfer in to 3rd tube.
- Repeat this same process up to 11th tube.
- Take two drop (or 100 µl) from 11th tube and discard it or save for further dilution if required.
- Add one drop (or 50 µl) 5% of 'O' blood group Rh (D) positive pooled red blood cells suspension in all tubes from 1st to 11th tubes.

- Mix gently all tubes and incubate at 37°C for 45 minutes.
- Also, follow the instruction of the blood centre SOP.
- Centrifuge at 1000 rpm for one minute and observe the agglutination.
- If there is no agglutination, wash the tubes three times with normal saline.
- Add two drops (or 100 μl) of AHG and mix gently, spin immediately at 1000 rpm for one minute and observe agglutination.
- If the titer shows 1-in-4 (agglutination grade 1+ or 2+) then we have to observe the tube 1-in-8 or 1-in-16 having no agglutination in the naked eye.
- The anti 'D' dilution which is showing 2+ reactions that dilution should be taken for preparation of sensitized red blood cells.

Example: If the titer 1:4 shows agglutination 2+ strength, then this dilution should be used for the preparation of check cell/ sentisitized cell.

Step II

- Take an equal volume of saline washed red blood cells and the desired titer of anti-D (agglutination of +2 strength).
- Incubate the tube at 37°C for one hour and mix the solution intermittently.
- Wash the sensitized red blood cells three times and prepare 5% of red blood cells suspension for utilization as required.
- To validate the sensitized red blood cells, we have to add AHG and observe the agglutination. If agglutination is present, then we confirm that the red blood cells are sensitized.

Practical Instruction of Sensitized Red Blood Cells Preparation

- First test tube which has only antisera and red blood cells suspension is called neat (Fig. 9.1). From 2nd tube to 11th tube according to serial number left-to-right direction

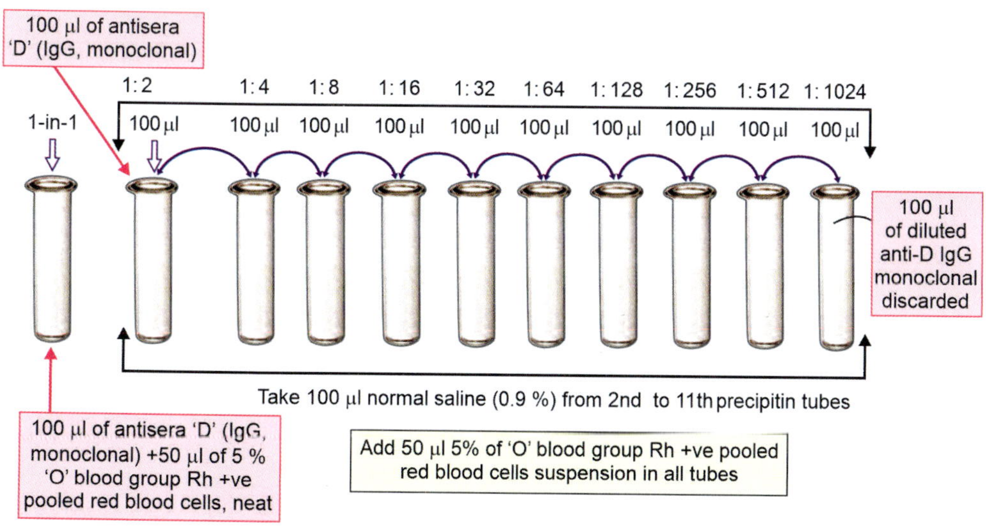

Fig. 9.1: Sensitized red blood cells preparation

titer is 1-in-2, 1-in-4, 1-in-8, 1-in-16, 1-in-32, 1-in-64, 1-in-128, 1-in-256, 1-in-512, 1-in-1024, respectively.
- Follow the above-mentioned steps about sensitized red blood cells preparation.

Follow the example as per requirement:

Preparation of 2 ml of sensitizing red blood cells:
- Take 0.8 ml normal saline + 0.2 ml antisera 'D' (IgG, monoclonal), (dilute the anti 'D' which is used) If 1 in 4 titers has shown 2+ agglutination. Add 1 ml 5% of 'O' blood group Rh +ve pooled red blood cells.
- Incubate the tube at 37°C for one hour and mix the solution intermittently.
- Wash the sensitized red blood cells three times and prepare 5% of red blood cell suspension for utilization as required.
- To validate the sensitized red blood cells, we have to add AHG and observe the agglutination. If agglutination is present, then we confirm that the red blood cells are sensitized.

Or

- To prepare 4 ml of sensitized red cells, take 3 ml normal saline + 1 ml antisera 'D' (IgG, monoclonal) (dilute the anti 'D' which is used) + 4 ml 5% of 'O' blood group Rh +ve pooled red blood cells suspension.

Or

- Take one precipitin tube and add one drop (or 50 µl) of antisera 'D', three drops or 150 µl of normal saline, the ratio is 1 in 4 and add four drops (or 200 µl) of prepared 5% of 'O' blood group Rh +ve pooled red blood cells suspension (50% of diluted anti 'D' + 50% of 'O' blood group Rh +ve pooled red blood cells suspension, ratio 50:50). Mix well.

Chapter 10

Coombs Test

Principle

The antihuman globulin (AHG) test was invented by Coombs. In 1945, Race and Mourant used AHG to detect antibodies over red cells or in the plasma and the test is called the Coombs test. It detects IgG type of antibody. Polyspecific (IgG + C_3d) AHG is used to detect both IgG and IgM (complement) type of antibodies. Coombs test is also known as the antiglobulin test. There are two types of tests.

- **Direct (DCT) or Direct antihuman globulin test (DAT):** It is the detection of sensitized red cells with IgG or *in vivo** sensitized cells. No serum is added to the cells, and no incubation is required.

  DAT is required to diagnose the following disease conditions:
  A. Hemolytic disease of the newborn (HDN)
  B. Autoimmune hemolytic anemias (AIHA)
  C. Drug-induced hemolytic anemias.
  D. Hemolytic transfusion reaction (HTR)
- **Indirect (ICT) or Indirect antihuman globulin test (IAT):** It is the detection of free antibodies present in the plasma or serum. Here, the pooled O cell is incubated with the plasma (in which the Ab is present). The pooled O cell is sensitised (*in vitro***) by the said antibodies. After washing the pooled O cell, AHG is added to the test, and observed for agglutination. The sensitised red cells show agglutination if Ab is present in the serum or plasma.

DIRECT ANTIHUMAN GLOBULIN TEST (DAT) THROUGH STANDARD TUBE TECHNIQUE

Reagents and Materials Required

1. Precipitin test tubes or standard glass test tubes.
2. Micropipette or pasture pipette.
3. Digital table top centrifuge machine.
4. Washed red blood cells suspension.
5. Antihuman globulin (AHG).
6. Bovine albumin (use for –ve control).
7. IgG-sensitized red cells (used for validity check).

**In vivo* means inside the body.

***In vitro* means outside the body, i.e. in the laboratory test.

Procedure

- Take two precipitin test tubes or standard glass test tubes and mark on the tubes as test and –ve control, respectively (Fig. 10.1).
- Take 2–3 drops of fresh blood to be tested in a test and negative control tube.
- Prefer fresh samples for testing and do not use the hemolysed red blood cell suspension for the DAT test.
- Wash the red blood cells of both the tubes (test and –ve control) 3–4 times in a large volume of normal saline to remove the unbound Abs or free globulin molecules.
- Completely decant the final supernatant wash.
- Refer to Chapter 3 for the steps to wash the red cells.
- Take two drops (or 100 µl) of antihuman globulin (AHG) into the tube marked as test.
- The negative control tubes are put along with the test.
- Take two drops (or 100 µl) of 6% of bovine albumin into the tube marked as –ve control.
- Prepare 6% from 22% of bovine albumin (1.4 ml 22% bovine albumin and 3.6 ml normal saline).
- Mix gently both the tubes (test and –ve control) and incubate at room temperature (20–24°C) for 2–5 minutes.
- Also follow the manufacturer's instructions documented in the literature.
- After incubation centrifuge at 1000 rpm for one minute and observe the agglutination macroscopically and microscopically.

Interpretation and Validity Check

- If agglutination is present in the test and no agglutination in the –ve control tube, it indicates that DAT positive and the test is valid.
- If no agglutination shows in both tubes, it indicates DAT negative.
- To rule out false negative results, all negative tubes should be re-tested by adding one drop (or 50 µl) of known IgG sensitized red cells (Coombs control red cells) and re-centrifuge at 1000 rpm for one minute. Immediately check for agglutination.
- If there is no agglutination found, that means the test is invalid and whole procedure should be repeated. If agglutination shows, the result is valid.
- If agglutination is observed in –ve control tube too then the test is invalid. Repeat the test.

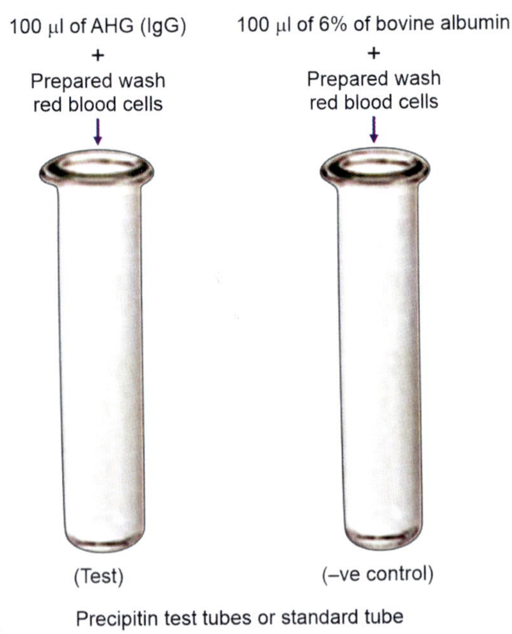

Fig. 10.1: Practical instruction for DAT

INDIRECT COOMBS TEST (IAT/ICT) THROUGH TUBE TECHNIQUE

Indication

- To detect incomplete antibodies during pregnancy.

- Compatibility testing.
- To detect Du antigen.
- To detect some antibodies against minor blood group antigens (antibody screening/identification)

Note: Antibody screening panel cell (2- or 3-cell panel) should be prefered over pooled O cell. Pooled O cell where the antigen profile is not known, can miss identification of an antibody if the antigen is not present in the pool. However, panel cells have almost all antigens of clinical significant.

Reagents and Materials Required

1. Pilot test tubes, precipitin test tubes or standard glass test tubes.
2. Micropipette or pasture pipette.
3. Digital table top centrifuge machine.
4. Digital display incubator
5. Test serum
6. 5% of 'O'Rh +ve and Rh –ve pooled red blood cells suspension.
7. Antihuman globulin (AHG)
8. Antisera 'D' IgG monoclonal (can use only IgG anti-'D' for IAT positive control: IgM will agglutinate it, so cannot use blend (IgG + IgM).
9. IgG-sensitized red blood cells (validity check)
10. 0.9% normal saline

Note: Pooled 'O' red blood cells suspension is prepared by taking pilot tubes from known 'O' blood group blood bags present in the inventory. Both 'O' positive and 'O' negative cells are taken for better antigenic expression (D, C, c, E, e) of polled cells for IAT (IgG) and also used for reverse grouping (IgM) reaction. A ratio of 3-in-1 (three Rh +ve and one Rh –ve having individual) pooled red cells is preferred.

PROCEDURE

- Take pilot test tube for preparation of 5% of confirm 'O' blood group pooled red blood cells suspension.
- Prefer fresh samples for testing and do not use the hemolysed red blood cells suspension for IAT test.
- Separate the test serum. It should be clear and free from hemolysis.
- Take three precipitin tubes or standard glass tubes for testing and mark on tubes as Test, +ve control and –ve control respectively.
- The positive and negative control tubes are put along with the test.
- Take two drops (or 100 µl) of patient serum in a test.
- Take two drops (or 100 µl) of antisera 'D' IgG monoclonal in a +Ve control tube.
- Do not use blend IgG + IgM antisera 'D' in a +ve control tube. (Blend IgG + IgM wille get agglutinate immediately after adding cells because of IgM).
- Take two drops (or 100 µl) of 6% of bovine albumin in a –ve control tube (prepared 6% from 22% of bovine albumin 1.4 ml 22% of bovine albumin and 3.6 ml normal saline).

- Add one drop (or 50 µl) of 5% prepared 'O' group wash pooled red blood cells suspension in a test, +ve control and –ve control tubes.
- Mix gently all the tubes—test and control.
- Incubate all the tubes at 37°C for one hour and also follow the manufacturer's instructions documented in the literature.
- After incubation, centrifuge at 1000 rpm for one minute. If any agglutination is detected, then it indicates the presence of saline phase antibody (IgM type).
- Examine for haemolysis and/or agglutination.
- If no agglutination or hemolysis is detected, then wash all the tubes (test and control tubes) 3–4 times in large volume of normal saline.
- Decant the supernatant fluid from the tubes in each wash as much as possible.
- After last wash add two drops (or 100 µl) of antihuman globulin (AHG) into the tubes marked as test, +ve and –ve control to the red cells button.
- Mix gently all the tubes (test and control) and centrifuge at 1000 rpm for one minute and observe the agglutination macroscopically and microscopically.
- Autocontrol should be kept with IAT.

  Keep +ve and –ve control for IAT.

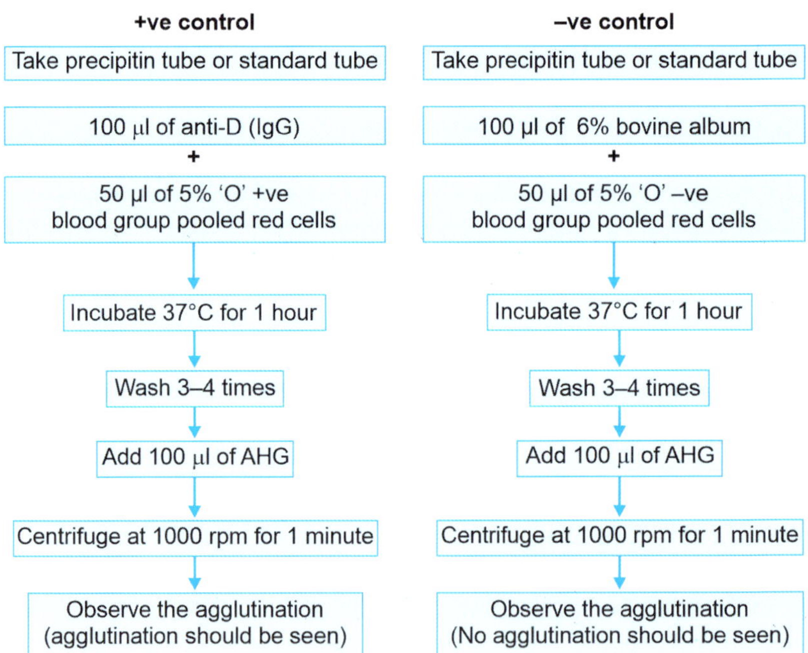

Interpretation and Validity Check

- If agglutination is there in tubes labelled as test and +ve control tube, no agglutination in the –ve control tube interprets as IAT positive.
- If no agglutination in test and –ve control tubes, indicates IAT is negative.
- If agglutination is present in –ve control tube, it may be due to autoagglutination.

- To rule out false negative results, all negative tubes should be re-tested by adding one drop (or 50 µl) of known IgG-sensitized red cells (Coombs control red cells) and re-centrifuge at 1000 rpm for one minute. Immediate check for agglutination.
- If there is no agglutination after adding check cell, then the test result is invalid and the whole procedure should be repeated. If agglutination is detected, then the result is valid.

Practical Instruction of IAT/ICT through Titration Technique

Step 1

- Take 11 precipitin test tubes or standard glass test tubes and arrange them serially in vertical position from left-to-right direction in a horizontal wooden rack (Fig. 10.2).
- Mark on the tubes 1st to 11th by marker. 1st tube is labelled as neat.
- Deliver two drops (or 100 µl) of normal saline (0.9%) using a standard pasture pipette or using micropipette from 2nd (labelled as 1 in 2) to 11th tubes leaving the 1st tube in this row, labelled as 1-in-2 to 1-in-1024.
- Add two drops (or 100 µl) of patient serum using a standard pasture pipette or using micropipette in 1st and 2nd tubes.
- Mix gently serum with saline in 2nd tube.
- Do not use the hemolysed serum.
- Take two drops (or 100 µl) of diluted sample from 2nd tube and transfer in to 3rd tube. Repeat this same process up to 11th tube. Take two drops (or 100 µl) from 11th tube and discard it or save for further dilution if required.
- Add one drop (or 50 µl) 5% of 'O' blood group Rh-positive and Rh-negative pooled red blood cells suspension (a ratio of pooled is 3-in-1) in all tubes from 1st to 11th tubes. Mix gently all the tubes from 1st to 11th and incubate at 37°C for 1 hour.
- Do not use the hemolysed red blood cell suspension.

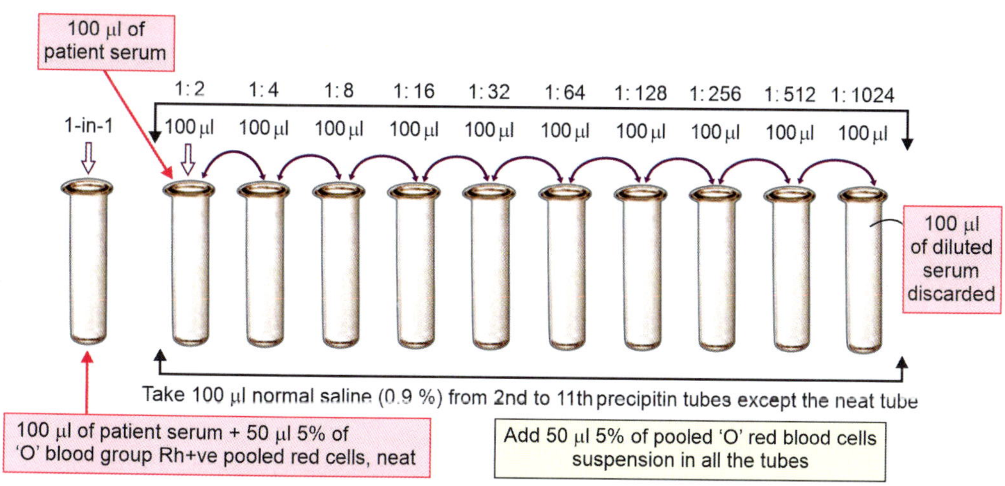

Fig. 10.2: IAT/ICT through titration

IAT/ICT through titration

- 1st test tube which has only serum and red blood cells suspension is called neat. From 2nd tube to 11th tube according to serial number left to right direction titer is 1-in-2, 1-in-4, 1-in-8, 1-in-16, 1-in-32, 1-in-64, 1-in-128, 1-in-256, 1-in-512, 1-in-1024, respectively.

Step 2

- After incubation, centrifuge at 1000 rpm for one minute.
- Examination for hemolysis and/or agglutination.
- If agglutination shows in the +ve control tube and no agglutination is observed test and negative control tubes.
- Washed all the tubes 3–4 times in a large volume of normal saline.
- Decant the supernatant fluid from the tubes in each wash as much as possible.
- Follow the above mention steps for red blood cell washing in Chapter 3.

Step 3 (After Last Wash)

Add 100 µl of antihuman globulin (AHG) in all the tubes including neat (Fig. 10.3).

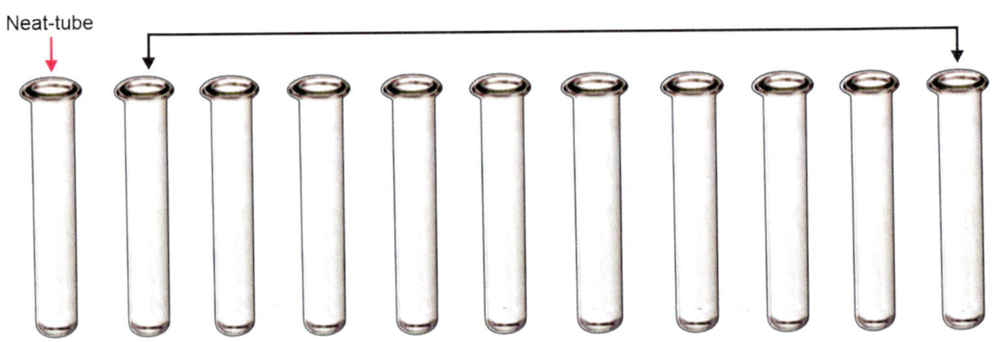

Fig. 10.3: Antihuman globulin reagent added in tubes

- Mix gently all the tubes and centrifuge at 1000 rpm for one minute and observe the agglutination macroscopically and microscopically and read the result from high titre to neat.

DAT AND IAT Test through Column Agglutination Technique (Gel Card)

Reagents/apparatus required

1. Coombs gel card (used for DAT and IAT test).
2. Reagent O cell (for IAT).
3. Readymade diluents (LISS solution).

And follow the same above-mentioned blood grouping instructions.

Step 1

Preparation 0.8–1% of red blood cells suspension (for DAT):

Take 1000 µl of readymade diluents (LISS solution) +10 µl of patient's packed RBCs in a precipitin tube. Mix gently.

Step 2

Remove aluminum foil of micro-tube in upright position of card.

Add 50 µl of the above red blood cells suspension to a pre-labelled micro-well on the Coombs card.

Step 3

Centrifuge the card in gel centrifuge machine for 10 mins.

Step 4

Follow the read results and grade the results accordingly above-mentioned instruction of blood grouping test (*see* Chapter 4).

IAT (Indirect Antiglobulin Test) through Column Agglutination Technique (Gel Card)

Step 1

Remove the aluminum foil micro-tube in the upright position of card.

Add 50 µl readymade-prepared are red blood cells pooled to a pre-labelled micro-well on the Coombs card (Fig. 10.4).

Step 2

Add 25 µl of patient plasma/serum to the gel micro-tube (prefer serum).

Step 3

Incubate the card at 37°C for 15 minutes.

Step 4

Centrifuge the card in a gel card centrifuge machine for 10 minutes.

Step 5

Read the results and grade the results accordingly as per the above-mentioned instruction of the blood grouping test (*see* Chapter 4).

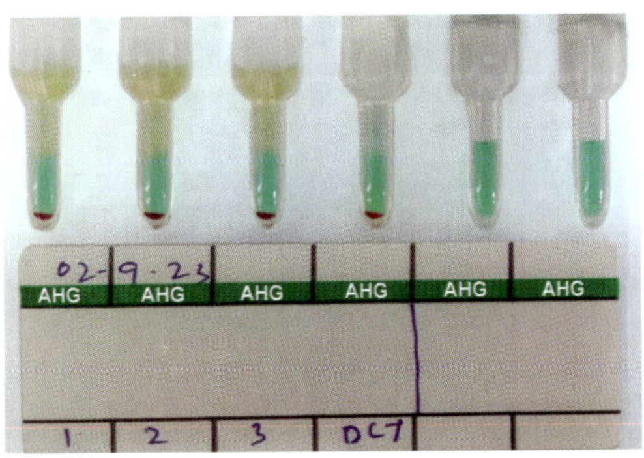

Fig. 10.4: DAT and IAT/antibody screening by gel card

Du TEST OR WEAK 'D' TEST THROUGH TUBE TECHNIQUE

Some red blood cells carry 'D' antigen that is expressed so weakly that the cells are not directly agglutinated by most anti 'D' sera used. It is Coombs indirect agglutination test (antihuman globulin test) done for weak antigens.

Reagents required

1. 2–5% of red blood cells suspension.
2. Anti 'D' (IgG, monoclonal, 1st choice) or blend (IgG + IgM) anti 'D'.
3. Antihuman globulin (AHG).
4. Bovine albumin.

Procedure

- Take a pilot test tube for preparation of red blood cells suspension and precipitin test tube or standard test tube for testing.
- Prepare 2–5% of red blood cell suspension of the blood to be tested (prefer 5% of red blood cell suspension for serological tube testing).
- Prefer fresh samples for testing and do not use the hemolysed cell suspension for Du test.
- Prepare 2–5% of confirm Rh +ve red blood cells suspension for +ve control.
- Prepare 2–5% of confirmed Rh –ve red blood cells suspension for –ve control.
- Take three precipitin tubes or standard glass tubes and mark on tubes as test, +ve control and –ve control respectively (Fig. 10.5).
- Take one drop (or 50 µl) of monoclonal IgG anti-D (1st choice) or blend (IgG + IgM) anti 'D' into the tube marked as test, +ve control and –ve control tubes.
- If anti 'D' (IgG, monoclonal) commercially is not available, blend (IgG + IgM) anti 'D' can be used.
- Add one drop (or 50 µl) of 2–5% prepared wash red blood cells suspension which test resulted 'D' negative on routine testing with anti 'D' into the tubes marked as test tubes. (Prefer 5% of red blood cell suspension for serological tube testing.)
- Add one drop (or 50 µl) of 2–5 % Rh +ve prepared to wash red blood cells suspension into the tube marked as +ve control tube, Rh–ve red cells as negative control tubes.
- The positive and negative control tubes are put along with the test.
- Mix gently all the tubes (test, +ve and –ve control) and incubate 37°C for 20–30 minutes and also follow the manufacturer's instruction documented in the literature.
- After incubation centrifuges all the tubes at 1000 rpm for one minute.
- Shake gently and observe the agglutination.
- If strong agglutination is observed only in the test tube and +ve control tube but not in the –ve control tube interprets as 'D' +ve and there is no need to proceed further.
- If no agglutination is observed test and –ve control tubes then wash the red blood cells 3–4 times in a large volume of normal saline.
- Decant the supernatant fluid from tubes as much as possible.
- Follow the above-mentioned steps about washing (*see* Chapter 3).
- Take two drops (or100 µl) of antihuman globulin in all the tubes (test, +ve and –ve control).
- Centrifuge all the tubes at 1000 rpm for one minute.
- Observe the agglutination macroscopically and microscopically.

Interpretation

- If agglutination shows in the test tube and +ve control tube but no agglutination in the –ve control tube it indicates the Du test is positive.
- If no agglutination shows in –ve control and test tubes it indicates Du test is negative.
- If agglutination is observed in –ve control tube too then it could be due to auto agglutination or due to a direct antiglobulin test (DAT) positive or invalid test.

PRACTICAL INSTRUCTION

Step 1

- Mix gently all the tubes (test, +ve and –ve control) and incubate 37°C for 20–30 minutes and also follow the manufacturer's instructions documented in the literature.
- Also follow the instruction of the blood centre SOP.
- After incubation, centrifuge all the tubes at 1000 rpm for one minute.
- Shake gently and observe the agglutination.

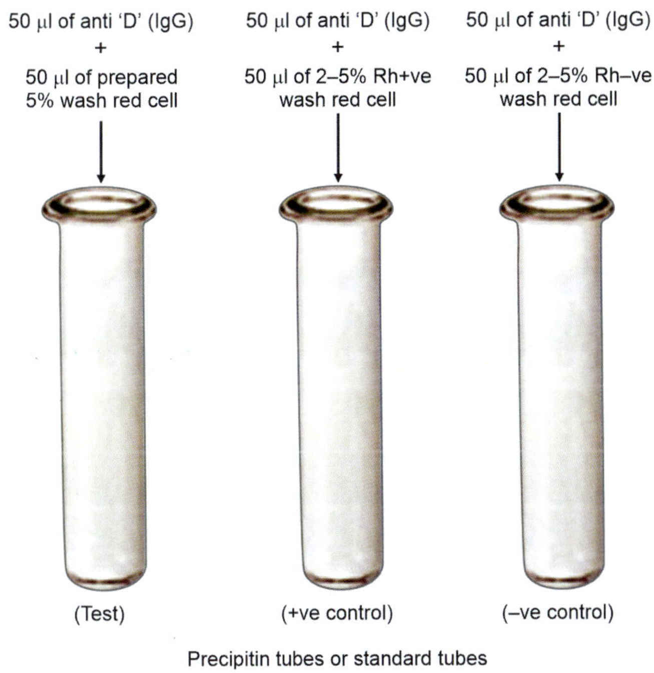

Fig. 10.5: Du test or weak 'D' test through tube technique

Step 2

- If no agglutination is observed test and –ve control tubes.
- Wash all the tubes (test, +ve and –ve control) three times with normal saline.
- Follow the above-mentioned steps about washing (*see* Chapter 3).
- Add two drops (or 100 μl) of antihuman globulin in all the tubes (test, +ve and –ve control). Centrifuge all the tubes at 1000 rpm for one minute. Observe the agglutination macroscopically and microscopically.

D^WEAK TEST THROUGH COLUMN AGGLUTINATION TECHNIQUE (GEL CARD METHOD)

Reagents/Apparatus Required

1. Coombs anti-IgG/LISS Coombs Gel card (Fig. 10.6).
2. Anti-D (IgG) for confirmation of D^{weak} by IAT.
3. Readymade diluents (LISS solution).

And follow the same above-mentioned blood grouping instructions.

Step 1

- Preparation 0.8–1% of red blood cells suspension.
- Take 1000 µl of readymade diluents (LISS solution) + 10 µl of patient's packed RBCs in a precipitin test tube. Mix gently.

Step 2

- Remove aluminium foil of micro-tube in upright position of card.
- Add 50 µl of above 0.8–1% of red blood cells suspension of samples to be tested for D^{weak} in 1 gel micro-tube of LISS Coombs/Coombs anti-IgG cards.

Step 3

Add 50 µl of anti-D (IgG) for confirmation of D^{weak} by IAT.

Step 4

Incubation for 15 minutes at 37°C.

Step 5

- Centrifugation for 10 minutes in gel card centrifuge machine.
- The result is interprited as per the agglution observed in the gel column.

Note: During D^{weak} determination, DCT for the same sample needs to be run simultaneously.

If DCT is positive, the RBCs need to be free from sensitization by suitable elution technique, then perform D^{weak} test. If agglutination is detected, the it is reported as weak D positive. The basic difference between RhD positive and weak D positive red cells is mentioned in Table 10.1.

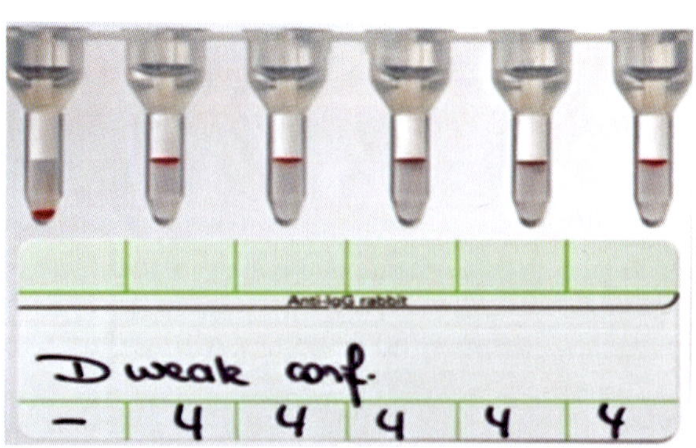

Fig. 10.6: D^{weak} test through column agglutination technique

Table 10.1: Reaction of Rh-D and Rh-D^{weak}		
Differentiation between Rh-D and Rh-D^{weak}	*Reactions*	*Reactions*
Direct test using a gel card with anti-D	++++	++ to negative
Confirmatory test with the gel card Coombs anti-IgG	++++	+++ to +
Results	Rh-D-Positive	Rh^{weak} D/DVI

Disinfection and cleaning protocol

Machine should be cleaned once in a week or in case of sample spillage.

Use soft cloths/cotton balls/gauze dipped in a mild soap solution (Dettol/Savlon) to wipe, clean the chambers of the incubator and rotor head centrifuge.

Chapter 11

Crossmatching/ Compatibility Testing

PRINCIPLE

The purpose of the crossmatch is to detect the presence of antibodies in the recipient against the red blood cells of the donor. These antibodies attach to the red blood cells of the donor after transfusion.

It detects the antibodies against the minor antigens present on donor red blood cells (RBCs), i.e. Duffy, Kell. Kidd, Lutheran, etc. which (Ags) are not typed routinely in blood centre. Crossmatching is the final test before issuing blood unit for transfusion.

i. Donor's red blood cells + Patient's serum = Major crossmatching (D)

ii. Patient's red blood cells + Donor's serum = Minor crossmatching (R)

Major crossmatching: This is one of the most important and routine procedures. In this procedure, we are looking for antibodies in the recipient against the donor red blood cells antigens. Therefore, we need serum from the recipient and red blood cells from the donor.

Minor crossmatching: It is not a routine procedure. These detect antibodies in the donor serum to the recipient's red blood cells. Therefore, for this we need serum from the donor and red blood cells from the recipient.

Auto-control: We also perform an auto-control with our crossmatches, i.e. recipient serum with recipient red blood cells suspension.

Types of Crossmatching

- **Saline crossmatch (IgM):** It is also known as the immediate spin method. In this method, other blood group system also reacts like M, N, Lewis^a and Lewis^b, P1 are detected. (Also follow the instruction of the blood centre SOP).
- **Coombs crossmatch (IgG) by indirect anti globulin test (IAT):** It is the commonly followed method of compatibility testing in almost all blood centres. The patient's serum is incubated with the donor red cell suspension at 37°C for one hour by conventional tubing technique (CTT). Wash three times and add AHG and centrifuge the tube to look for agglutination. In this method, the antibodies (IgG type) against minor blood group systems like Rh system like D, c, E, C, e; also Ss, Fy^a and Fy^b, Jk^a and Jk^b, Kell, Lu^a and Lu^b is detected.
- Follow the instruction of the blood centre SOP.
- **Enzyme crossmatch (IgG) by papain cysteine enzyme:** Similar to AHG method, additional enzyme is added to the serum, donor cell suspension. Enzyme enhances

the antigenic expression of Rh system (C, c, D, E, e). Proteolytic enzymes digest the cell membrane and expose the antigens, which react with IgG antibodies and thus bring out compatibility more clearly.

- Increases reactivity to Rh, Jk, P1, Le and I antibodies.
- Removes certain antigens e.g. M, N, S, Fy^a and Fy^b.
- So, enzyme methods will help in differentiating multiple allo-antibodies.
- Follow the instruction of the blood centre SOP.
- **Enzyme crossmatch (IgG) by bovine albumin:** It takes 45 minutes by tube method. In this method, other blood group systems like Ss, Fy^a and Fy^b, Jk^a and Jk^b, Kell, Lu^a and Lu^b and Rh system like C, c, D, E, e also reacts.
- Follow the instruction of the blood centre SOP.

Column Agglutination Technique (Gel Card Method) (Crossmatching and Antibody Screening)

Advantages of Column Techniques (IgG)

- The column agglutination technique is simple, reliable, rapid to use, and very sensitive. Column technique can be used for any immunohematological test such as ABO and Rh typing, DAT, IAT, other blood group systems, antibody identification, and crossmatching. After testing, it can preserve for a long time as a record. The specific kit available consists of a small tube filled with about 35 µl cephadex gel and Coombs reagent.

1. SALINE CROSSMATCH (IgM) THROUGH TUBE METHOD

Reagents/Apparatus Required

1. Two pilot test tubes (12 × 100 mm) and two precipitin test tubes or standard test tubes.
2. Test tube rack/wooden rack.
3. Micropipette or pasture pipette.
4. Digital display incubator.
5. Digital bench-top centrifuge machine.
6. 2–5% of red blood cell suspension for both donor and recipient.
7. Donor and recipient serum.
8. 0.9% of normal saline.

- Take two pilot test tubes and prepare 2–5% of red blood cell suspension for both donor and recipient separately (Fig. 11.1). Prefer fresh samples for testing and do not use the hemolysed red cell suspension for the saline crossmatch test.
- Take two precipitin test tubes or standard glass test tubes and mark on tubes as test 'D' for major crossmatch and 'R' for the minor crossmatch.
- To the tube marked as 'D' add two drops (or 100 µl) of recipient serum and one drop (or 50 µl) of prepared donor red blood cells suspension.
- To the tube marked as 'R' add two drops (or 100 µl) of donor serum and one drop (or 50 µl) of 2–5% prepared recipient red blood cells suspension (prefer 5% of red blood cells suspension for serological tube testing).
- Donor and recipient serum should be clear and free from hemolysis.
- Mix well both the tubes ('D' and 'R') and incubate 5–10 minutes at room temperature and also follow the manufacturer's instruction documented in the literature.

- Follow the instruction of the blood centre SOP.
- After incubation centrifuge both the tubes at 1000 rpm for one minute (in an emergency, it can be centrifuged without any incubation and termed as immediate spin crossmatch) and observe the agglutination or hemolysis macroscopically and microscopically.

Result:

Agglutination = Incompatible

No agglutination = Compatible

Practical Instruction

- Mix well both the tubes ('D' and 'R') and incubate 5–10 minutes at room temperature.
- Follow the instruction of the blood centre SOP.
- After incubation centrifuge both tubes at 1000 rpm for one minute and observe the agglutination or hemolysis macroscopically and microscopically.

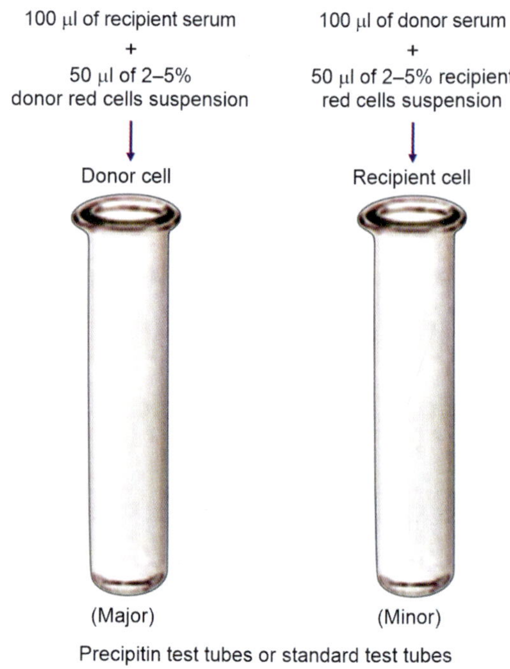

Fig. 11.1: Saline crossmatch (IgM) through tube method

Result:

Agglutination = Incompatible

No-agglutination = Compatible

Interpretation

Saline crossmatch (IgM) test tube.

1. **Agglutination:** IgM type antibody (ant-M, anti-N),

   ABO incompatibility: Rule out clerical error.
2. **No agglutination:** Absence of IgM antibody.

   It does not rule out IgG type of antibody. So, risk of delayed hemolytic transfusion reaction is there.
3. Saline crossmatch (IgM) test tube should be incubated at room temperature but sometimes the blood group systems like M, N, P1, Lea and Leb may also react 37°C (IgG). So AHG crossmatches are required to identify this (IgG) type of antibody.

Crossmatching Testing in Emergencies through Tube Method

On the request of the clinician, blood can be issued on an emergency basis, after blood grouping and Rh typing followed by crossmatch by saline method (IgM).

Steps are followed as mentioned in the saline crossmatch skipping the step of incubation. Both major and minor crossmatch tubes should be spin immediately at 1000 rpm for one minute and observe the agglutination or hemolysis macroscopically and microscopically.

In extreme cases, where there is no time to take a sample and to test it, O-Rh(D) negative blood, preferably red cells, may be transfused with the request of the clinician and consent from patient party.

Donor unit that has not been tested or partially tested for compatibility for IgM and IgG antibodies against patient's serum, should be clearly labelled 'uncrossmatched blood'.

2. COOMBS CROSSMATCH/IAT (IgG) THROUGH TUBE METHOD USING ANTIHUMAN GLOBULIN (AHG)

IAT crossmatching helps to rule out any antibody (IgG) present in the serum. There is no requirement for any control run during IAT crossmatching.

Autocontrol is run in every crossmatch when there is an incompatibility due to the autoantibody.

- All the above-mentioned reagents, and apparatus used for saline crossmatching, and AHG are needed in IAT crossmatching.
- Prepare 5% of red blood cells suspension for both donor and recipient.

Step 1

- Take two pilot test tubes and prepare 5% of red blood cell suspension for both donor and recipient (Fig. 11.2).
- Prefer fresh samples for testing and do not use the haemolysed red blood cell suspension for IAT crossmatch test.
- Take two precipitin test tubes or standard glass test tubes and mark on tubes as test 'D' for major crossmatch and 'R' for minor crossmatch.
- To the tube marked as 'D' take two drops (or 100 µl) of recipient serum and one drop (or 50 µl) of prepared 5% donor red blood cells suspension.
- To the tube marked as 'R' take two drops (or 100 µl) of donor serum and one drop (or 50 µl) of prepared 5% recipient red blood cells suspension.
- Donor and recipient serum should be clear and free from hemolysis.
- Mix well both the tubes ('D' and 'R') and incubate at 37°C for one hour.
- Also follow the instructions of the blood centre SOP.

Step 2

- After incubation, wash all the tubes 3–4 times in large volume of normal saline.
- Decant the supernatant fluid from tubes thoroughly.
- After the last wash, add two drops (or 100 µl) of antihuman globulin (AHG) into the tubes marked as donor and recipient ('D' and 'R') to the red cells button.
- Centrifuge both tubes at 1000 rpm for one minute and observe the agglutination or hemolysis, macroscopically and microscopically.

Practical Instruction

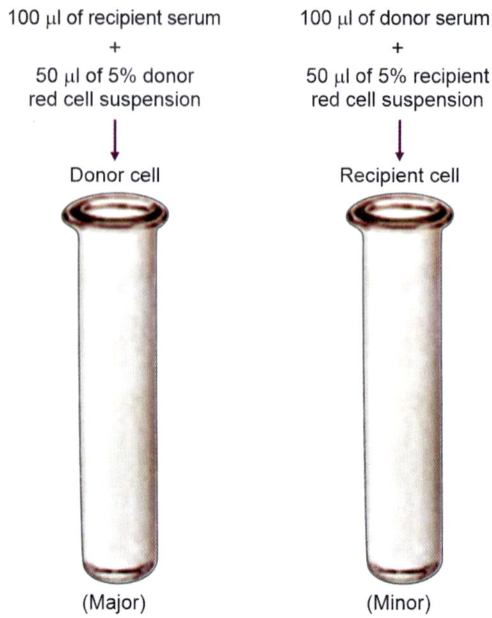

Fig. 11.2: Coombs crossmatch/IAT (IgG) through tube method

Result:

Agglutination = Incompatible

No agglutination = Compatible

Crossmatching through Column Agglutination Technique (Gel Card) (IgG)

Reagents/Apparatus Required

1. Two pilot test tubes and two precipitin test tubes or standard test tubes.
2. Micropipette.
3. Digital display incubator.
4. Crossmatching LISS/coombs gel card.
5. Digital bench top gel centrifuge machine.
6. 0.8–1% red blood cells suspension for both donor and recipient.
7. Donor and recipient serum/plasma.
8. Diluents (LISS solution).

Procedure

- Take two pilot test tubes and prepare wash packed red blood cells suspension for both donor and recipient separately.
- Advantage of CAT is that washing step is not required.
- Prefer fresh samples for testing and do not use the hemolysed red blood cells suspension for column agglutination (gel card) crossmatch test.
- Take two precipitin test tubes or standard test tubes and mark on tubes as test 'D' for major crossmatch and 'R' for minor crossmatch.

- Prepare 1% of red blood cells suspension for donor and recipient.
- To the tube mark as 'D' (major) take 1000 µl of LISS solution and 10 µl from prepared donor packed red blood cells.
- To the tube mark as 'R' (minor) take 1000 µl of LISS solution and 10 µl from prepared recipient packed red blood cells. Mix gently both the tubes.
- Take gel card and mark on card as test 'D' for major crossmatch and 'R' for minor crossmatch and name of patient or patient ID for major and minor crossmatch.
- Remove aluminium foil of micro-tube in upright position of card.
- Take 50 µl of prepared 1% of red blood cells suspension from 'D' tube and charge on gel LISS/Coombs card at 45° angle marked 'D' and add 25 µl of recipient serum at 90° angle.
- Serum should be clear and free from hemolysis.
- Similarly, take 50 µl of prepared 1% red blood cells suspension from 'R' tube and charge in gel LISS/Coombs card at 45° angle marked 'R' and add 25 µl of donor serum at 90° angle.
- Autocontrol—pipette 50 µl of 1% of recipient red blood cells suspension in a micro-tube and add 25 µl of recipient serum/plasma in a micro-tube.
- Incubate 37°C for 15 minutes and also follow the manufacturer's instruction documented in the literature.
- After incubation centrifuge 1176 rpm for 10 minutes in gel centrifuge machine and also follow the manufacturer's instruction documented in the literature.
- Follow the instruction mentioned in the blood centre SOP. Routinely only patient serum (25 µl) is tested with the donor cell (50 µl) for crossmatching.
- Observe the result.
- If red blood cells settle at the bottom, then it is compatible.
- It is defined as incompatible, if red cells float or retained in the gel column
- The strength of agglutination is depicted as 1+ to 4+ (Fig. 11.3)

Interpretation

- **No agglutination:** If there is no agglutination, then the donor unit is compatible. There is no detectable antibody in the patient's plasma.
- Crossmatch compatible can be possible if the antibody titer is very low or the antigens on the red cell is of single dose (heterozygous).
- **Agglutination:** There is presence of Ab against the donor red cells.

  The patient should be transfused with Ag-negative donor red cell.

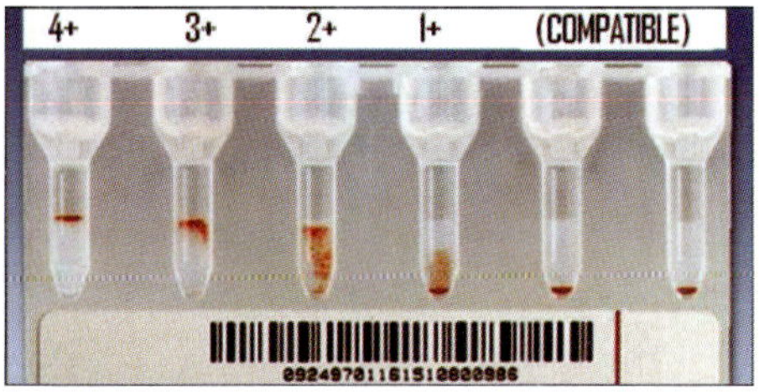

Fig. 11.3: Crossmatching through column agglutination technique (gel card) (IgG): Showing various grades of agglutination (incompatibility) and compatible crossmatch (last 2 columns)

Antibody screening should be done in multi-transfused patients and if there is history of alloantibody, then the patient should be transfused with Ag-negative blood unit even if the antibody screening is negative.

3. ENZYME CROSSMATCH (IgG) BY PAPAIN CYSTEINE ENZYME BY TUBE METHOD

Follow the same above-mentioned saline crossmatching reagent and apparatus and extra papain cysteine enzyme reagent needed in enzyme crossmatching.

- Take two pilot tubes and prepare 2–5% of red blood cell suspension for both donor and recipient separately (Fig. 11.4).
- Prefer fresh samples for testing and do not use the hemolysed red cells suspension for enzyme crossmatch test.
- Take two precipitin tubes or standard glass tubes and mark on tubes as test 'D' for major crossmatch and 'R' for minor crossmatch.
- To the tube marked as 'D' take two drops (or 100 µl) of recipient serum and add one drop (or 50 µl) of papain cysteine enzyme and one drop (or 50 µl) of 2–5% prepared donor red blood cells suspension (prefer 5% of red blood cells suspension for serological tube testing).
- To the tube marked as 'R' take two drops (or 100 µl) of donor serum add one drop (or 50 µl) of papain cysteine enzyme and one drop (or 50 µl) of prepared recipient red blood cells suspension.
- Donor and recipient serum should be clear and free from hemolysis.

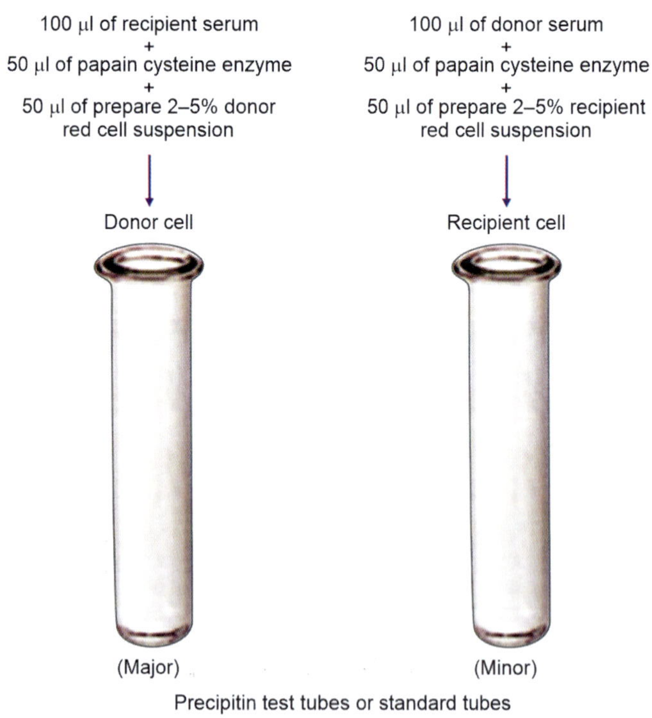

Fig. 11.4: Enzyme crossmatch (IgG) by papain cysteine enzyme by tube method

- Mix well both the tubes ('D' and 'R') and incubate 37°C for 45 minutes and also follow the manufacturer's instruction documented in the literature.
- Also follow the instruction of the blood centre SOP.
- After incubation centrifuge both tubes at 1000 rpm for one minute and observe the agglutination or haemolysis macroscopically and microscopically.

Result

Agglutination = Incompatible

No agglutination = Compatible

4. ENZYME CROSSMATCHING (IgG) BY BOVINE ALBUMIN THROUGH TUBE METHOD

- Follow the above-mentioned saline crossmatching steps. Extra bovine albumin enzyme reagent is needed in enzyme crossmatching.
- Prepare 2–5% red blood cell suspension for both donor and recipient.
- Take two pilot tubes and prepare 2–5% of red blood cell suspension for both donor and recipient separately (Fig. 11.5).
- Prefer fresh samples for testing and do not use the hemolysed red blood cell suspension for the bovine albumin crossmatch test.
- Take two precipitin test tubes or standard glass test tubes and mark on tubes as test 'D' for major crossmatch and 'R' for minor crossmatch.
- To the tube mark as 'D' take two drops (or 100 µl) of recipient serum and one drop (or 50 µl) of 6% of bovine albumin on top of the serum (albumin should be from a layer on top of the serum. Do not mix).
- Take one drop (or 50 µl) of prepared 2–5% donor red blood cells suspension so as to form a layer on top. (Now, there are three layers in the tube.)

  Prefer 5% of red blood cell suspension for serological tube testing.
- Serum should be clear and free from hemolysis.
- To the tube marked as 'R' take two drops (or 100 µl) of donor serum and one drop or 50 µl of 6% bovine albumin on top of the serum (albumin should from a layer on top of the serum. Do not mix).
- Take one drop (or 50 µl) of prepared 2–5% recipient red blood cells suspension so as to form a layer on top. (Now, there are three layers in the tube.)

  (Prefer 5% of red blood cell suspension for serological tube testing).
- Incubate it at 37°C for 15 to 30 minutes.
- After incubation centrifuge both tubes at 1000 rpm for one minute and observe the agglutination or hemolysis macroscopically and microscopically.
- Also follow the instruction of the blood centre SOP.

Result

Agglutination = Incompatible

No agglutination = Compatible

Practical Instruction

Step 1

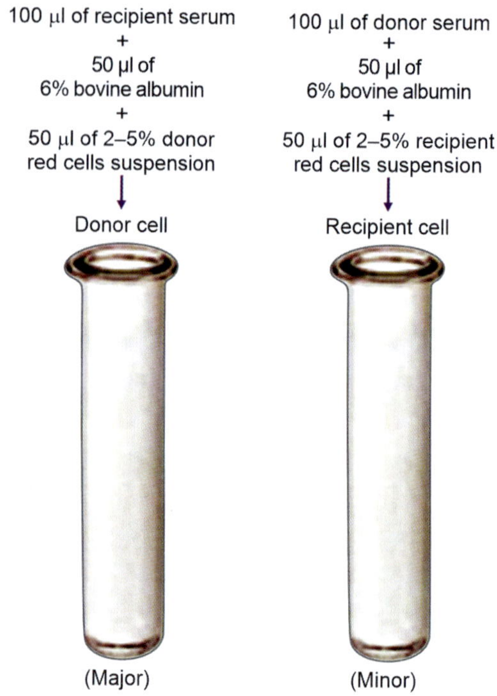

Fig. 11.5: Enzyme crossmatching (IgG) by bovine albumin through tube method

Step 2

- Incubate it at 37°C for 15 to 30 minutes.
- After incubation centrifuge both tubes at 1000 rpm for one minute and observe the agglutination or hemolysis macroscopically and microscopically.

Result

Agglutination = Incompatible

No agglutination = Compatible

Note:
- If antibody screening using panel cell (R1R1, R2R2, rr) for both recipient and donor unit is found to be negative, then minor crossmatching is not required.
- Minor crossmatching is only done for issuing plasma to pediatric patients or whole blood.
- The major crossmatch is used to detect unexpected blood group antibodies in patient's serum against antigens on donor red blood cells. Positive reaction in any test indicates incompatibility.

Interpretation of IgM and IgG Crossmatch

Anti 'A' and anti 'B' are IgM type of antibody and can be detected in saline/bovine/immediate spin crossmatch. Other minor antibodies like Rh, Kell, Duffy, Kidd, MNS are IgG type of antibody and detected by AHG crossmatch.

Cause of Hemolytic Transfusion Reaction

ABO-incompatible transfusion which is mostly due to clerical error or misdentification of patient, leads to immediate hemolytic transfusion reaction. This can be prevented by saline crossmatch.

IgG type of antibodies which are mostly against the minor blood group Ags like Rh, Kell, duffy, and Kidd, are responsible for delayed hemolytic transfusion reaction. This can be prevented by AHG crossmatching and transfusing Ag matched blood units.

NB: Routinely minor crossmatch is not performed.

Chapter 12

Crossmatching Protocol for Exchange Transfusion in a Case of HDFN

PRINCIPLE

- For patients with known hemolytic diseases of fetus and newborn (HDFN) close observation of bilirubin levels and "Hemoglobin" is warranted to determine whether there is a need for neonatal exchange transfusion to remove bilirubin and maternal antibody.
- Exchange transfusion is the use of whole blood or equivalent to replace the neonate's circulating blood and simultaneously remove maternal antibodies and bilirubin.
- The blood unit should be compatible with both maternal serum and baby.

Materials Required

- Table top centrifuge.
- 37°C incubator.
- LISS-Coombs gel cards (column agglutination technique).
- Dedicated 37°C incubator for column agglutination.
- Dedicated gel card centrifuge machine.
- Micropipette, pasture pipettes, test tubes, beakers and filter paper.
- Automated cell counter to determine the hematocrit level.
- Sterile connecting device.
- Leuko-filter for PRBC.
- Transfer bag.
- Wafers (to join two different bags).
- 0.9% normal saline.

Reagents

- Antisera (anti-A, anti-B, anti-AB, anti-D_1 and D_2).
- Antihuman Globulin (anti-IgG + C_3d).
- 5% pooled red blood cell suspension (ABO) (reverse grouping of mother's sample (serum) and donor's plasma.
- Papain-cystein enzyme (maternal serum and donor's plasma should be screened for any irregular antibody through pooled 'O' cells and 'O' cells + papain cysteine enzyme).

Specimen

- Anticoagulated and clotted blood sample of the patient and his/her mother.
- Donor's blood sample (segment of donor PRBC and FFP unit).

Protocol for Double Volume Exchange Transfusion (DVET) in Newborns

- Newborn baby and mother's blood sample both are required for cases of neonatal jaundice for DVET.
- For transfusion purposes in neonates, both mother's and baby's samples are required, as the babies do not have any naturally occurring antibodies (anti-A/anti-B) in their serum up to 3–4 months of their life.
- Compatibility test is performed with both the mother's sample and the baby's sample.

Rule of thumb: ABO and Rh compatible blood is issued to the baby (must be compatible to both mother and baby).

PROCEDURE

- Centrifuge the sample of patient (both anticoagulated and clotted blood) at 3000 rpm for five minutes.
- A blood unit should be crossmatched against mother's serum by indirect coombs test (IAT/ICT), i.e. AHG phase testing.
- The blood unit should not be more than 5 to 7 days old.
- If maternal serum is having any allo-antibody, then the unit should be negative of the antigen against which the maternal antibody is directed.

> ***Example:*** If anti-E is identified in the mother's serum then the PRBC should be E antigen negative.

- Perform the minor crossmatch by column agglutination technique with the baby's cells and donor's compatible plasma or AB group plasma unit (neutral plasma) to ensure no transfusion reaction.
- If the crossmatch is incompatible, do antibody screening/identification to find the antibody. If the crossmatch is compatible then leuko reduction is performed using the leuko-filter. Lab-side filter/in-line filter is preferred over the bedside filter.
- After filtration, take a small volume of filtered PRBC (about 1 ml) and determine the HCT of that filtered blood.
- Calculate the amount of plasma to be added with the filtered PRBC to maintain the HCT level is between 45% and 50% by using the formula $C_1 V_1 = C_2 V_2$.
- Using a sterile connecting device, join both the bags of PRBC and FFP and transfer the required volume of FFP to the packed cell.
- Mix thoroughly and after mixing, take a small amount of that re-constituted blood and estimate the HCT.
- If the result of HCT is within the desirable range, you can issue that re-constituted blood.

Crossmatching through Column Agglutination Technique (Gel Card/IgG)

- Prepare 0.8–1% of red blood cells suspension of the donor and recipient.
- Choose a donor blood that is ABO compatible with mother and baby and antigen negative.

- To the tube mark as 'D' (major) take 1000 µl of LISS solution and 10 µl from the washed red cells of the donor unit.
- To the tube marked as 'R' (minor) take 1000 µl of LISS solution and 10 µl from prepared recipient red blood cells.
- Take a gel card and mark on the card as test 'D' for a major crossmatch and 'R' for a minor crossmatch.
- Remove the aluminium foil of the micro-well in the upright position of the card.
- Take 50 µl of prepared 1% of red blood cells suspension from 'D' tube and charge on gel LISS/Coombs card at 45° angle the micro-well marked 'D' and add 25 µl of mother's serum at 90°angle.
- Similarly, take 50 µl of prepared 1% red blood cells suspension from 'R' tube and charge in gel LISS/Coombs card at 45° angle the micro-well marked 'R' and add 25 µl of 'AB' group plasma or compatible plasma at 90° angle.
- Incubate 37°C for 15 minutes and also follow the manufacturer's instruction documented in the literature.
- After incubation centrifuge 1176 rpm for 10 minutes in gel centrifuge machine and also follow the manufacturer's instruction documented in the literature.

Coombs crossmatch/IAT (IgG) through tube method by antihuman globulin test (AHG)

- Follow the above-mentioned same crossmatching technique (IAT (IgG) for HDFN by CTT method (chapter 11).
- For major crossmatch 100 µl of mother's serum +50 µl of donor red cells. For minor crossmatch 100 µl of compatible plasma +50 µl of baby's red cells. Follow the remaining steps are same as that of Coombs crossmatch.

INTERPRETATION

- Absence of agglutination or hemolysis is a negative test result and indicates a serologically compatible crossmatch. This result should be interpreted as 'compatible'.
- Hemolysis or agglutination indicates a serologically incompatible crossmatch. This result is interpreted as 'incompatible''.
- In such case, obtain full details of patient, repeat the test on an additional fresh sample, and perform requisite test in consultation with the transfusion medicine doctor and treating doctor.
- For a case of HDFN crossmatching of blood units should be carried out under the supervision of a transfusion medicine specialist and continuous follow-up with the treating doctor.

Selection of Blood for Double Volume Exchange Transfusion

- Do the ABO and Rh grouping of both baby and mother.
- Select a unit which is compatible with both baby and mother as mentioned in Table 12.1.

Table 12.1: Selection of blood unit for double volume exchange transfusion in different blood group patients

Baby's blood group	*Mother's blood group*	*Blood selected for exchange transfusion*
' A' group	'A' group 'B' group 'AB' group 'O' group	'A' gr. 1st choice ('O' gr. 2nd) 'O' group 'A' gr. 1st choice ('O' gr. 2nd) O' group
'B' group	'A' group 'B' group 'AB' group 'O' group	'O' group 'B' gr. 1st choice ('O' gr. 2nd) 'B' gr. 1st choice ('O' gr. 2nd) 'O' group
'A B' group	'A' group 'B' group 'AB' group 'O' group	'A' gr. 1st choice ('O' gr. 2nd) 'B' gr. 1st choice ('O' gr. 2nd) 'AB' gr. 1st choice (A, B, O gr 2nd) 'O' group
'O' group	'A' group 'B' group 'AB' group 'O' group	'O' group 'O' group 'O' group 'O' group
Rh-positive	Rh-negative	Rh-negative
Rh-negative	Rh-positive	Rh-negative

Chapter 13

Transfusion Support in Autoimmune Hemolytic Anemia (AIHA)

- Antibodies are directed against one's own RBC that are called autoagglutinin or autoantibody.
- In the case of AIHA, the autoantibody which reacts with the corresponding antigen on the own red cells and causes hemolysis.
- Autoagglutinins not only react with own cells during cell typing, but also interfere with antibody screening/identification and crossmatching.
- Depending on the etiology, AIHA can be classified as primary (idiopathic) or secondary to NHL, CLL infection, and autoimmune diseases like SLE, Thymoma, and Sjogren syndrome.
- AIHA is also classified as warm, cold, or mixed type according to the thermal reactivity of autoagglutinins (as shown in Fig. 13.1). AIHA mainly presented with symptoms of anemia and laboratory findings of high or increased reticulocyte count, raised indirect bilirubin, LDH and positive DAT.
- Autoagglutinins react with most of the donor red cells when present in the serum of the patient. For patients suffering from AIHA, try to select a least incompatible unit by performing titration crossmatch by saline, enzyme, and AHG along with autocontrol.
- The compatibility test depends upon the specificity of the antibody. If a non-specific antibody is present, crossmatch with multiple donor units, by carrying out crossmatching using titration method (as given in Rh section). Issue incompatible blood (means using different panel of cells) for which titer is lowest.

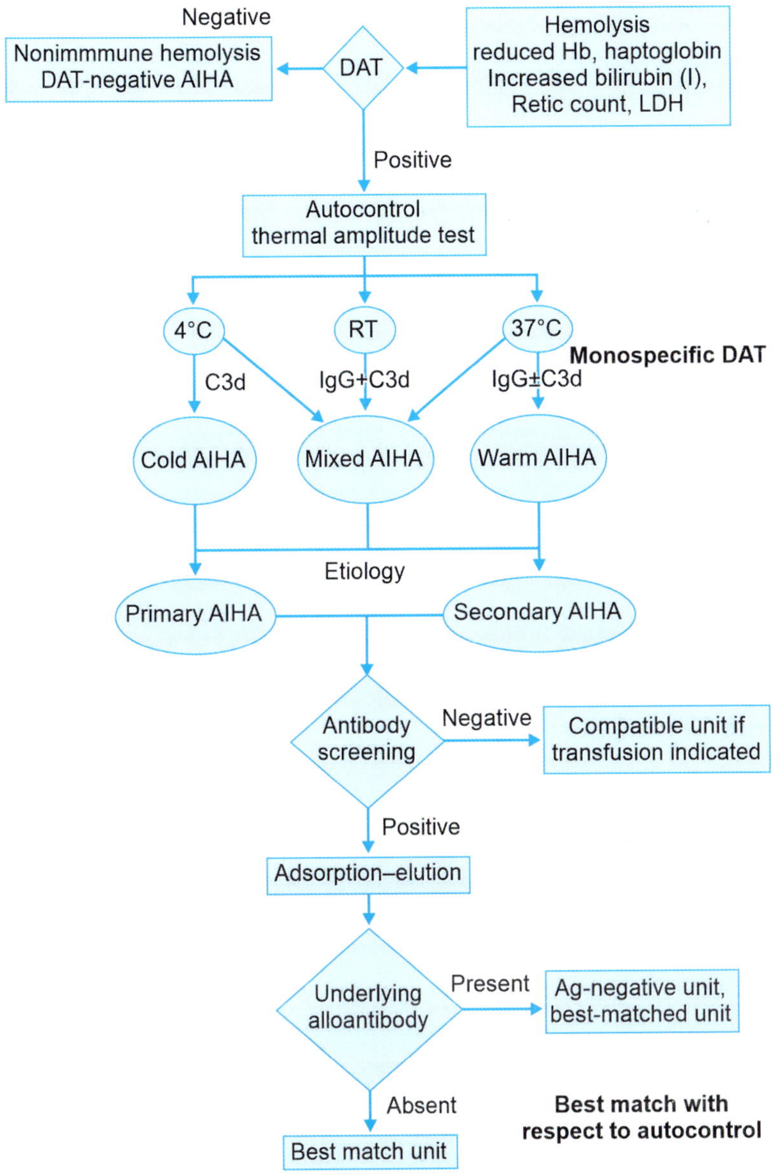

Fig. 13.1: Showing the diagnosis of AIHA and selection of best-match unit for transfusion

Selections of Least Incompatible Donor or Best-matched Unit through Cross-matching Procedures like Saline, Enzyme and IAT by Titration Method

1. Prepare serial twofold dilutions of the patient's serum or plasma. The dilution range should be from 1-in-2 to 1-in-1024.
2. Mix 2 drops of each dilution with 1 drop of a 3–5% cell suspension of red cells.

Reagents/Apparatus required

1. Two pilot test tubes and 44 precipitin test tubes or standard glass test tubes.
2. Wooden rack and test tube rack.

3. Micropipette or pasture pipette.
4. Digital display incubator.
5. Digital bench top centrifuge machine.
6. 2–5% of donor red blood cells suspension (for saline and enzyme method).
7. 5% of donor red blood cells suspension (for IAT)
8. Recipient serum.
9. Papain cysteine enzyme
10. Antihuman globulin (AHG).
11. 0.9% of normal saline.

Procedure

Similar to the conventional AHG crossmatching, crossmatch 4–6 units of donor RBC with the serum of an AIHA patient along with the autocontrol. The strength of agglutination of the crossmatch is compared with the autocontrol. The unit is considered as least incompatible or best match unit which has the strength of agglutination less than that of autocontrol.

NB: For cold autoantibodies, the compatibility is done both at 4°C and 37°C by means of titration method (issue the least incompatible blood). For a case of autoimmune hemolytic anemia (AIHA) transfusion should be carried out under the supervision of transfusion medicine and treating doctor.

Serial Dilution Titration Technique for Case of AIHA through Tube Method

Donor no. 01

- Take two pilot test tubes and prepare 2–5% of donor red blood cells suspension for saline and enzyme crossmatch (prefer 5% of red blood cells suspension for serological tube testing).
- For IAT crossmatch, prepare 5% of donor red blood cells suspension.
- Prefer fresh samples for testing and do not use the hemolysed red blood cells suspension or serum for case of AIHA crossmatch test.
- Take 44 precipitin test tubes or standard glass test tubes for saline, enzyme and IAT titration.
- Mark on the tubes from 1 to 11th titration for saline crossmatch and arrange the tubes in 1st row (incubate 4°C, IgM).
- Then another 1 to 11th titration for saline crossmatch arrange the tubes in 2nd row from left-to-right direction in horizontal wooden rack.
- Similarly, for enzyme crossmatch titration arrange the tubes from 1 to 11th in 3rd row.
- For IAT crossmatch titration 11 tubes are required and arrange them from 1 to 11th in 4th row.
- The first row should be kept in incubation at 4°C but the remaining three rows must be in incubation at 37°C.
- Deliver two drops (or 100 µl) of normal saline (0.9%) using standard pasture pipette, micropipette from all 2nd (labelled as 1-in-2) to 11th tubes in 1st, 2nd, 3rd and 4th row (total 40 tubes)

- Leaving the 1st tube in each row (total 4 tubes labelled as neat).
- Add two drops (or 100 µl) of recipient serum in 1st and 2nd tubes of 1st, 2nd, 3rd and 4th rows (Total 8 tubes).
- Mix gently serum with saline in 2nd tube of 2nd, 3rd and 4th rows (total 4 tubes).
- Take two drops (or 100 µl) diluted serum from 2nd tube of 1st row and transfer into 3rd tube. This process is to be done up to 11th tube. Discard two drops (or 100 µl) diluted serum from 11th tube or save for further dilution if required.
- Similarly take two drops (or 100 µl) diluted serum from 2nd tube of 2nd row and transfer into 3rd tube. This process is to be done up to 11th tube. Discard two drops (or 100 µl) diluted serum from 11th tube or save for further dilution if required.
- Similarly, follow in 3rd row from 2nd tube take two drops or 100 µl diluted serum and transfer into 3rd tube. This process is to be done up to 11th tube. Discard two drops (or 100 µl) diluted serum from 11th tube or save for further dilution if required.
- Similarly, follow in 4th row from 2nd tube take two drops (or 100 µl) diluted serum and transfer in to 3rd tube. This process is to be done up to 11th tube. Discard two drops (or 100 µl) diluted serum from 11th tube or save for further dilution if required.
- Add one drop (or 50 µl) of papain cysteine enzyme in 1st to 11th tube of 3rd row for enzyme crossmatching.
- Add one drop (or 50 µl) 2–5% of corresponding donor red blood cells suspension in all the tubes from 1st to 11th in 1st, 2nd and 3rd rows (total 33 tubes) for saline and enzyme crossmatching (prefer 5% of red blood cells suspension for serological tube testing).
- Similarly, add one drop (or 50 µl) 5% of corresponding donor red blood cells suspension in all the tubes from 1st to 11th in 4th row for IAT crossmatching.
- 1st tube of 1st, 2nd and 4th rows have only serum and corresponding donor red cells suspension but 1st tube of 3rd row has serum, papain cysteine enzyme and corresponding donor red blood cells suspension. All these tubes are called neat.
- From 2nd to 11th tube according to serial number left-to-right direction titer ratio is 1-in-2, 1-in-4, 1-in-8, 1-in-16, 1-in-32, 1-in-64, 1-in-128, 1-in-256, 1-in-512, 1-in-1024, respectively.
- Mix gently all test tubes (total 44 tubes) and keep 11 tubes form 1st rows are kept incubate at 4°C for 45 minutes (IgM). And the 2nd rows are kept incubate at 37°C for 45 minutes (IgM). And 3rd rows are kept incubate at 37°C for 45 minutes (IgG). The tubes of 4th row should be kept incubate at 37°C for one hour (IgG) and also follow the manufacturer's instruction documented in the literature. Also follow the instruction of the blood centre SOP.
- Centrifuge the tubes of 1st, 2nd and 3rd rows at 1000 rpm for one minute and read the titer.
- After incubation of 4th-row tubes, washed all the tubes 3–4 times in large volume of normal saline.
- Follow the above-mentioned steps for cell washing (*see* Chapter 3).

- After last wash add two drops (or 100 µl) of antihuman globulin (AHG) into the all tubes including neat tube to the red cell button.
- Centrifuge all the tubes at 1000 rpm for one minute and observe the titer or haemolysis macroscopically and microscopically.
- Similarly, follow the above-mentioned titration technique for other remaining donors and select the least incompatible donor for safe transfusion.

Practical Instruction

Master dilution titration technique through tube method for AIHA case:

- Take 33 test tubes (three sets, 11 tubes in each set) and labeled as mentioned in Fig. 13.2.
- Transfer 100 µl of diluted serum into each tube.
- Add 50 µl of red cell suspension of donor cell/pooled O cell.
- For saline crossmatch, keep one set room temperature for 45 minutes.
- For enzyme crossmatch, add 50 µl of enzyme and keep one set in incubator at 37°C for 45 minutes.
- For IAT crossmatch, keep one set in an incubator at 37°C for 45 minutes.
- After incubation, centrifuge the test tubes at 1000 rpm for 1 minute and observe for agglutination.
- For the last two sets of tubes, wash for three times, decant the supernatant completely and add 100 µl AHG. Then centrifuge and observe for agglutination
- All transfusion services should follow the definite protocol.
- Many centre follow the principle of 'best match' PRBCs in AIHA (Fig. 13.3). Here, routine crossmatch is compared with autocontrol and if the strength of agglutination is less than autocontrol, then it is considered as 'best match' or 'least incompatible' unit.

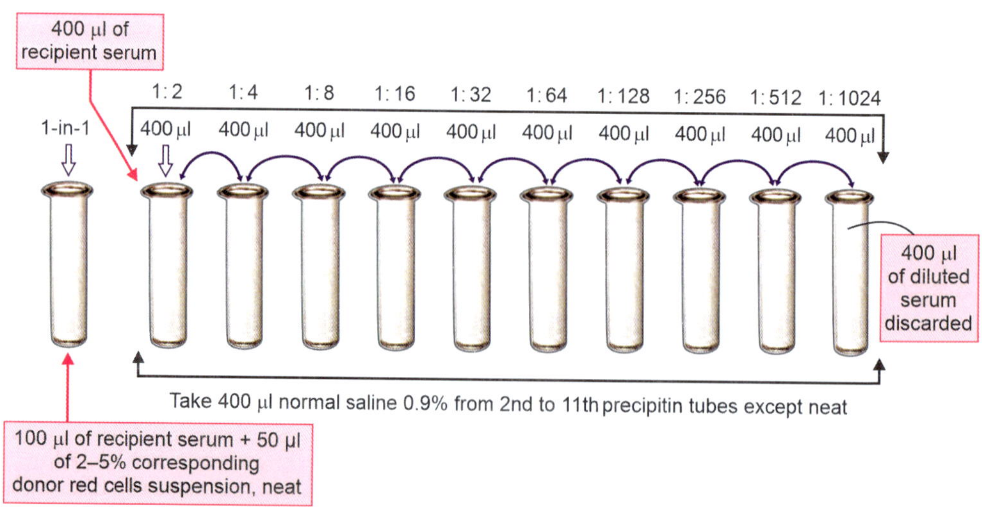

Fig. 13.2: Antibody titration (master dilution) of autoantibody

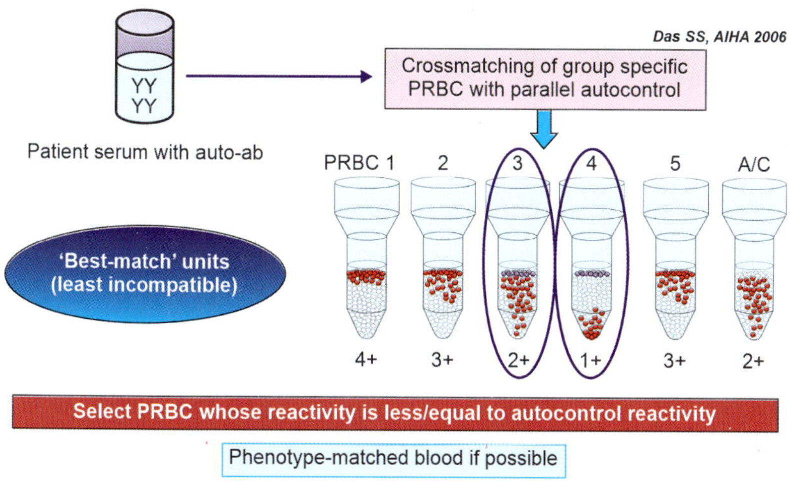

Fig. 13.3: Selection of best-match blood unit for AIHA patient

IMPORTANT MESSAGE

- IgM and IgG methods crossmatching are very much important to avoid transfusion reactions in multitransfused patients like AIHA, thalassemia, aplastic anemia, leukemia, cancer, renal failure, septicemia, ABO and Rh HDN, open heart surgery, transplantation, etc.
- Compatible 'O' negative packed red blood cells can be considered for transfusion on emergency basis.
- Gel technique is the best method for the case of AIHA. Donor units should be crossmatched in gel card in parallel with the DAT and autocontrol. The unit showing agglutination strength less or equal to the strength of reaction observed in autocontrol can be issued for transfusion under medical supervision.

Chapter 14

Preparation and Standardization of Papain Cysteine Enzyme and Anti-A_1 Lectin

Papain cysteine enzyme is used for antibody screening and enzyme crossmatching.

Principle

The papain cysteine enzyme preparations used in blood centre differ from lot to lot; each time a stock enzyme, solution is prepared, its reactivity should be tested and incubation periods standardized for optimal effectiveness.

The reaction of certain blood group antigen and antibodies are selectively enhanced by the use of enzymes. The enzymes enhance antibody reactivity to Rh, Kidd, P, Lewis and I antigens and destroy or depress reactivity to red cells antigens Fy^a, Fy^b, M, N, S.

PREPARATION TECHNIQUE

For 100 ml of papain cysteine reagent preparation weigh 1 g of papain purified powder (Lobacheme Pvt. Ltd.) and 0.485 g of L-cysteine hydrochloride (HS CH_2 CH (NH_2) COOH. HCl, Lobacheme).

Preparation of Phosphate Buffer Solution (Stock Solution)

1. M/15 $Na_2HPO_4.2H_2O$ (disodium hydrogen phosphate) 11.866 g/1000 ml of distil water.
2. M/15 KH_2PO_4 (potassium dihydrogen phosphate) 9.066 g/1000 of distill water.
3. Both these stock solutions are kept separately in two different bottles.

Phosphate buffer solution is prepared using these above reagents and the pH is adjusted to 7.4 either using NaOH or HCl.

For 100 ml of papain cysteine enzyme preparation take 80 ml of Na_2HPO_4 (4 volumes) + 20 ml of KH_2PO_4 (1 volume) in a beaker, mix well and adjust the pH 7.4.

[If prepared working phosphate buffer pH becomes <7.4, than add 5 (N) NaOH (10 g of NaOH in 50 ml of distill water) drop-by-drop and adjust the pH 7.4].

(If prepared buffer pH becomes >7.4, than add conc. HCl or diluted 1% HCl drop-by-drop and adjust the pH 7.4).

Preparation of Papain Cysteine Reagent

From prepared working buffer solution take 80 ml in a beaker and add 1 g of papain powder and mix well. Take 20 ml of buffer solution in separate beaker and add 0.485 g of L-cysteine hydrochloride and mix well.

Mix both the solutions in a beaker and filter with Whatman's filter paper and check the pH 6.2. Incubate the prepared solution at 37°C for one hour and again check the pH 6.2.

Standardize of prepared papain cystin enzyme by performing titration and specificity test.

Reagents/Apparatus Required

1. Two pilot test tubes and 11 precipitin test tubes or standard glass test tubes.
2. Wooden rack and test tube rack.
3. Micropipette or pasture pipette.
4. Digital table top centrifuge machine.
5. Digital display incubator.
6. 2–5% of 'O' blood group pooled red blood cells suspension.
7. Anti-'D' (IgG, monoclonol).
8. Papain cysteine enzyme.
9. 0.9% of normal saline.

Check the Strength of Papain L-cysteine Enzyme through Titration Method

- Take 11 precipitin test tubes or standard glass test tubes and arrange serially on vertical position from left-to-right direction in horizontal wooden rack (Fig. 14.1).
- Mark on the test tubes 1st to 11th by marker. 1st tubes labelled as neat.
- Deliver two drops (or 100 µl) of normal saline (0.9%) using standard pasture pipette or using micropipette from 2nd (labelled as 1-in-2) to 11th tubes leaving the 1st tube in this row, labelled as 1-in-2 to 1-in-1024.
- Add two drops (or 100 µl) of anti 'D' (IgG) using standard pasture pipette or using micropipette in 1st and 2nd tubes.
- Mix gently normal saline and anti 'D' (IgG) in the second tube.
- From 2nd tube take two drops (or 100 µl) of diluted anti 'D' (IgG) and transfer it into the third tube. This process is done up to 11th tube. From 11th tube two drops (or 100 µl) of anti-D is discarded or saved for further dilution if required.
- Add one drop (or 50 µl) of prepared papain cysteine enzyme in each tube from 1st to 11th tubes.
- Add one drop (or 50 µl) 2–5% of 'O' blood group pooled red blood cells suspension in all tubes from 1st to 11th tubes (prefer 5% of red blood cells suspension for serological tube testing).
- Do not use the hemolysed red blood cells suspension.
- Mix gently all tubes and incubate at 37°C for 45 minutes.
- After incubation centrifuge at 1000 rpm for one minute.
- And read the titer result macroscopically and microscopically.

PRACTICAL INSTRUCTION

Titration of anti-'D' (IgG).

STRENGTH OF PAPAIN CYSTEINE ENZYME THROUGH TITRATION METHOD

- 1st test tube which has only anti 'D' and cell suspension is called neat. From 2nd tube to 11th tube according to serial number left-to-right direction titer is 1-in-2, 1-in-4, 1-in 8, 1-in-16, 1-in-32, 1-in-64, 1-in-128, 1-in-256, 1-in-512, 1-in-1024, respectively.

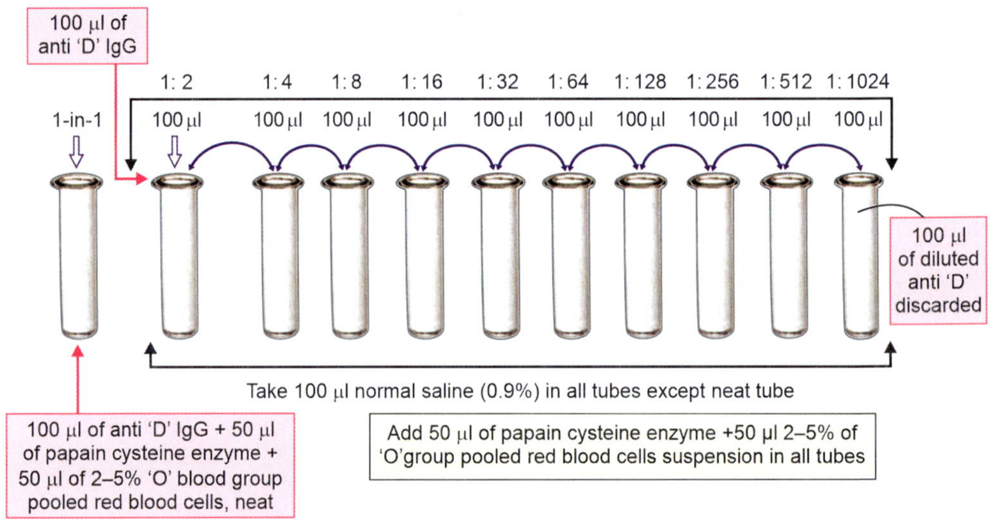

Fig. 14.1: Strength of papain cysteine enzyme through titration

> **Note:**
> 1. If agglutination of titer anti 'D' shows 1:16 or above, i.e. your papain cysteine enzyme preparation is correct.
> 2. If commercial prepared papain cysteine enzyme and laboratory prepared enzyme are same in anti 'D' (IgG) titer then the preparation is correct.

SPECIFICITY TEST

Follow the above-mentioned reagent and apparatus of papain enzyme titration, extra 10 pilot tubes for cells suspension preparation of different known corresponding blood group 2–5 % of pooled red blood cells needed in specificity test (prefer 5% of red blood cells suspension for serological tube testing).

Practical Instruction

Take 50 μl of papain cysteine enzyme in each tube and add different known corresponding blood group 2–5% 50 μl of pooled red blood cells suspension

- Mix gently anti 'D' IgG and red blood cells suspension in all the tubes from 1st to 10th and incubate at 37°C for 45 minutes and centrifuge in 1000 rpm for one minute.
- Observe the result for specificity test (Fig. 14.2).

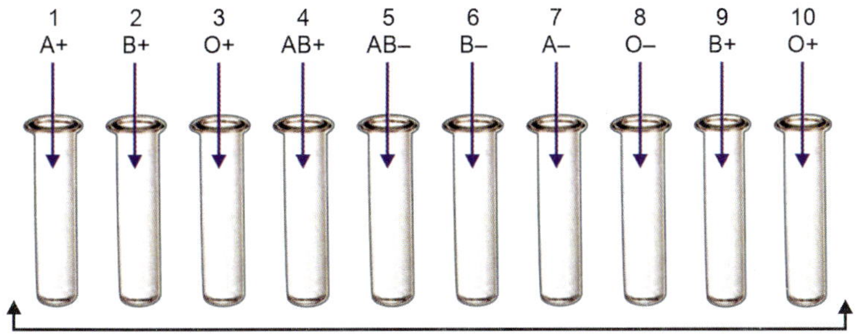

Fig. 14.2: Strength of papain cysteine enzyme through titration

Note:

1. After preparation of papain cysteine enzyme store in aliquot small sterile vial at –20°C to –40°C in deep freeze.
2. Do not keep used enzyme in deep freeze because of interfering prozone phenomena.

Preparation and Standardization of Lectin Dolichos Biflorus (A_1)

Principle

Saline extracts of seeds react with specific carbohydrates on red blood cells membranes and make useful typing reagents that are highly specific at appropriate dilutions.

Diluted extract of dolichos biflorus agglutinates A_1 red blood cells but not A_2 red blood cells.

Uses of anti 'A_1 lectin: For classification of 'A' subgroups ('A_1', 'A_2' and 'A_1B', 'A_2B').

Reagents Preparation

Seeds may be obtained from health-food stores, pharmacies or commercial seed companies.

The seeds should be raw.

Add 10 g of seeds (Kuthi Dal) in 100 ml of normal saline or 5 g of seeds in 50 ml of normal saline in a beaker.

1. Grind the seeds in a food processor or crush the seeds with the help of mortar and pestle.
2. Soak seeds in a sterile normal saline in a large test tube or small beaker, place ground seeds and three to four times their volume of saline. (Seeds vary in the quantity of saline they absorb.) Incubate at room temperature for 4 to 12 hours, stirring or inverting occasionally. Or at 4°C blood keeping refrigerator for overnight.
3. Centrifuge 'hard spin' at 5000 rpm for 5–10 minutes.

Transfer supernatant reagent in another separate tube and again centrifuge for clear supernatant.

Check pH 7.0.

Dolichos Biflorus ('A_1' Lectin Extract)

Test dilutions of the extract to find dilution for the desired activity. Determine the activity of the extract with the appropriate red blood cells, as bellow:

A. Add one drop (or 50 µl) of 2–5% normal saline suspension of known 'A_1', 'A_2' 'A_1B' 'A_2 B', 'B' and 'O' red blood cells to appropriately labelled tubes.

B. Add one drop (or 50 µl) of A_1 lectin extract to each tube.

C. Centrifuge for calibrated time.

D. Inspect for agglutination and record results.

E. The A_1 lectin should agglutinate 'A_1' and 'A_1 B' blood group red blood cells, but not 'A_2', 'A_2 B', 'B', and 'O' blood group red blood cells.

The native extract often agglutinates all the red blood cells tested. To make the product useful for reagent purposes, add enough saline to the extract so that there is 3+ or 4+ agglutination of 'A_1' and 'A_1B' red blood cells, but not 'A_2', 'A_2 B', 'B', and 'O' red blood cells.

Do the titration with pooled A_1 and A_2 blood group red blood cells suspension.

Test for the specificity with different 20 blood group red blood cells suspension.

Test dilutions of the extract to find the dilution for the desired activity. Determine the activity of the extract with the appropriate red cells.

Titration method:

- Take 11 precipitin test tubes or standard glass test tubes and arrange serially on vertical position from left-to-right direction in horizontal wooden rack in 1st row for A_1 cells (Fig 14.3).
- Take 11 precipitin test tubes or standard glass test tubes and arrange serially on vertical position from left-to-right direction in horizontal wooden rack in 2nd row for A_2 cells.
- Mark on the test tubes 1st to 11th by marker. 1st tube labelled as neat for A_1 and A_2 cells.
- Deliver two drops (or 100 µl) of normal saline (0.9%) in 1st and 2nd row using standard pasture pipette or using micropipette from 2nd (labelled as 1-in-2) to 11th tubes leaving the 1st tube in this row, labelled as 1-in-2 to 1-in-1024.
- Add two drops (or 100 µl) of anti 'A_1' lectin using standard pasture pipette or using auto pipette in 1st and 2nd tube of 1st and 2nd row.
- Mix gently normal saline and anti 'A_1' lectin in second tube of 1st and 2nd row.
- From 2nd tube take two drops (or 100 µl) of diluted anti 'A_1' lectin and transfer into third tube this process done up to 11th tube (1st and 2nd row). From 11th tube two drops (or 100 µl) discard it or save for further dilution if required.
- Add one drop (or 50 µl) 2–5% of 'A_1' blood group pooled red blood cells suspension in all tubes from 1st to 11th in 1st row.
- Add one drop (or 50 µl) 2–5% of 'A_2' blood group pooled red blood cells suspension in all tubes from 1st to 11th in 2nd row.

  (Prefer 5% of pooled red blood cells suspension for serological tube testing).

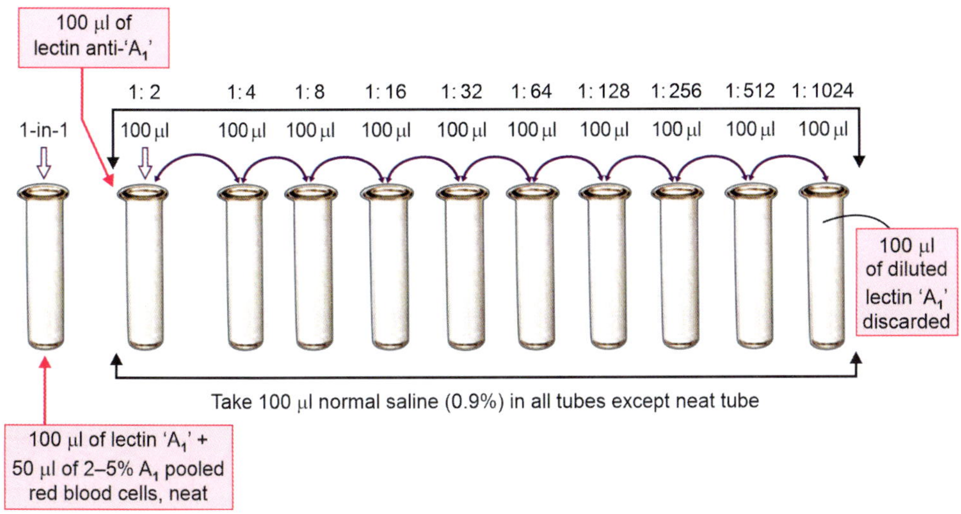

Fig. 14.3: Anti 'A_1' lectin titration using A_1 red blood cell

- Do not use the hemolysed red blood cells suspension.
- Mix gently all tubes and incubate at room temperature (20 to 24°C) for 45 minutes.
- After incubation centrifuge at 1000 rpm for one minute.
- And read the titer result macroscopically and microscopically.

Similarly follow the above-mentioned titration technique for other remaining blood groups like 'A_1B', 'A_2B', 'B' and 'O' red blood cells.

If titer result shows 1-in-16, use A_1 lectin reagent for test.

If titer shows high 1-in-64 or 1-in-128, then dilute the reagent with normal saline and the ratio should be 1-in-4 or 1-in-8).

After dilution check the A_1 lectin reagent with 'A_1' group red blood cells and use the reagent for test.

- The titration results should be read from lesser concentration to higher concentration.

Practical Instruction

Check the strength of anti 'A_1' lectin through A_1 red blood cell.

Add 50 µl of 2–5% of 'A_1' blood group pooled red blood cells suspension in all tubes.

- Add 100 anti-A_1 lectin to the neat test tube and 2nd test tube labelled as 1:2.
- From 2nd tube to 11th tube according to serial number left to right direction titer is
- 1-in-2, 1-in-4, 1-in-8, 1 in 16, 1 in 32, 1 in 64, 1-in-128, 1-in-256, 1-in-512, 1-in-1024, respectively.
- Add 50 µl of 2–5% of 'A_2' blood group pooled red blood cells suspension in all tubes.

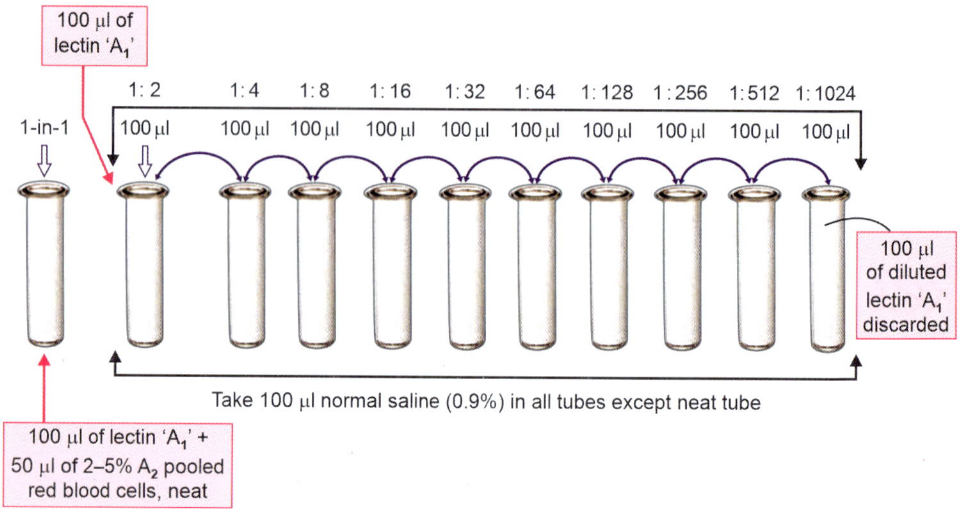

Fig. 14.4: Anti 'A_1' lectin titration using A_2 red cell

Result:

A_1 red cells titer shows 1-in-16

A_2 red cells titer shows negative.

Specificity Test of A_1 Lectin through Tube Method

Practical Instruction

- Add 100 µl of anti-A_1 lectin in each tube and add different known corresponding blood group 2–5% of 50 µl of pooled red blood cells suspension (Fig. 14.4).

Mix gently anti 'A_1' lectin and red blood cells suspension in all the tubes from 1st to 10th and incubate at room temperature for 45 minutes and centrifuge in 1000 rpm for one minute. Also follow the instruction of the blood centre SOP.

- Observe the result for specificity test (Fig. 14.5).
- After preparation of anti-A_1 lectin extract store in aliquot small sterile vial at –20°C to –40°C in deep freeze.

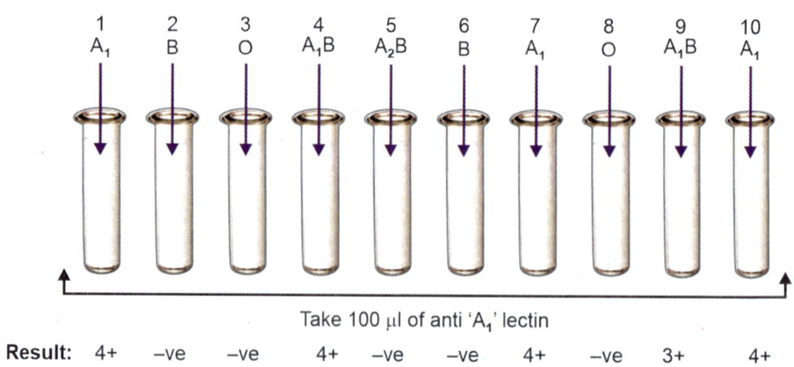

Fig. 14.5: Specificity test of A_1 lectin through tube method

Chapter 15

Quality Control of Antisera and Reagent Red Cells

Quality control (QC) is the management of the testing process:

- Reagents must be tested to determine if they have maintained their specificity and sensitivity.
- The quality control should be done to check new batches to ensure that they comply with all biological standards.
- A vial from each new batch/lot should be checked for its appearance, specificity, avidity, reactivity, and potency (titer) using known positive and negative control.
- Appearance, specificity, and avidity of reagents should be checked daily.
- There should be no reaction with negative control, no cross-reactive, and no rouleaux or prozone phenomena.
- The reagent should be clear on visual inspection daily.
- No reagents should be used after the date of expiry.
- It is the responsibility of the senior technician (technical supervisor) in the immunohematology laboratory to ensure the quality of reagents.
- Daily quality control checks and lot QC should be performed along with proper documentation.
- This quality control has to be carried out every month and for each new lot.
- All antisera must be complying with all the quality control criteria as mentioned in Drug and Cosmetic Act/DGHS.
- All blood grouping and antihuman globulin (AHG) reagents should be kept in refrigerators at 2°C–6°C. The manufacturer's instructions should be followed for storage.
- All reagents should be clearly labelled with the batch number, expiry date, and storage temperature.
- All reagents should be used according to the manufacturer's instructions.
- They must be re-standardized if they are to be used by alternative techniques or in a diluted form (e.g. ABO and Rh typing in microplates or automatic system).
- New reagents should not be issued for routine testing until quality control has done and validated that the new reagents are satisfactory.

QUALITY CONTROL OF REAGENT RED CELLS

- Reagent red cells should be prepared daily from a minimum pool of 3–5 individual cells for each group (A, B, and O).
- A pool of reagent red cells should be washed at least 3 times with normal saline and 1% or 5% cell suspension is prepared as per CAT or CTT testing method.
- Quality requirements for reagent red cells (Table 15.1).

Table 15.1: Quality control of reagent red cell		
Parameters	*Quality requirement*	*Frequency*
Appearance	No hemolysis or turbidity in the supernatant by visual inspections	Daily
Reactivity and specificity	Clear cut reactions with known sera against red blood cells antigens	Each day
	Anti-A Anti-B	
	A cell 4+ 0 B cell 0 4+ O cell 0 0	

QUALITY CONTROL OF REAGENT ANTISERA

- **Appearance:** The antisera reagent should be clear on visual inspection. There should be no turbidity, precipitate or gel formation, discolouration and no particles observed in the antisera reagent vial.
- **Specificity:** It denotes that antisera reagent should react only with red cells having the corresponding antigen while it should not react with other antigens on red cells. For specificity testing, the antisera reagent should be tested with three different red cells of the corresponding antigen and three different red cells, which lack the corresponding antigen (Table 15.2).

Table 15.2: Quality control of reagent antisera					
Antisera	*A cell*	*B cell*	*O cell*	*RhD positive cell*	*RhD negative cell*
Anti-A	4+	0	0		
Anti-B	0	4+	0		
Anti-D				4+	0
AHG	Reactive with Coomb's control cell Negative with O cell				

- **Avidity:** It is the time (in seconds) taken by the antibodies to show the first agglutination. The test is done by mixing two drops of anti-serum with one drop of 40–50% cell suspension on a slide at room temperature (RT). A stop watch is used to record the time for a visible reaction (+1) and then for a strong (+4) reaction to occur (Table 15.3).

Table 15.3: Quality control: Avidity of different antisera					
Type of cells used	A_1	A_2	A_2B	*B*	*O*
Anti-A	3 to 4 seconds	5 to 6 seconds	5 to 6 seconds	Negative	Negative
Anti-B	Negative	Negative	5 to 6 second	3 to 4 seconds	Negative
Anti-D	RhD positive		RhD negative		
	5 to 10 seconds		Negative		

- **Reactivity:** It denotes that antisera should not cause immune hemolysis due to excessive antibodies (prozone phenomenon) when it reacts with the corresponding antigen. It also shows that there should not be rouleaux formation by antisera due to excessive protein contents.
- **Potency (titer):** Titer is defined as the highest dilution of antibodies at which it shows visible agglutination. It checks the capacity of antisera to react with the corresponding antigen in serial dilution. Undiluted antisera should give the highest reaction strength, while with serial dilution, reaction strength should decrease gradually.

PRACTICAL ORIENTATION FOR QUALITY CONTROL OF ANTISERA AND REAGENT RED CELLS

Serial Dilution Titration Technique through Standard Tube Method

Quality Control of ABO Reagents

The main criteria for the quality of ABO antibody reagents are testing for specificity, and potency (avidity, and titer). There should be no reaction with negative control, no cross reactivity and no rouleaux or prozone phenomena.

The reagent should be clear on visual inspection daily.

Reagents/apparatus Required

1. Pilot test tubes and 44 precipitin test tubes or standard glass test tubes.
2. Horizontal wooden rack and test tube rack.
3. Micropipette or pasture pipette.
4. Digital table top centrifuge machine.
5. 0.9% normal saline.
6. Antisera 'A', 'B' and 'AB' (monoclonal)
7. 5% of 'A'_1', 'A'_2', 'B', 'A_1 B', and 'A_2B' pooled red blood cells suspension.

TITRATION

- **Titration of antisera:** 5% of corresponding antigen containing pooled red blood cells suspension (blood group Rh + Ve or Rh – ve) is used for titration of antisera checking.

  A antigen pooled red blood cell suspension (A_1, A_2, A_1B and A_2B) are used for antisera 'A' (IgM) titer.

  B antigen pooled red blood cell suspension (B, A_1B and A_2B) are used for antisera 'B' (IgM) titer.

  A and B antigen pooled red blood cell suspension (A_1, A_2, A_1 B, A_2B and B) are used for antisera 'AB' (IgM) titer.

  'O' blood group pooled red blood cell suspension is used for antisera 'H' lectin titer (Bombay group).

  'A_1' blood group pooled red blood cells is used for antisera A_1 lectin titer.
- Take 44 precipitin test tubes or standard glass test tubes for titration of antisera 'A', 'B' and 'AB'.
- Mark on the tubes from 1 to 11th (e.g. 1:1, 1:2 to 1:1024) titration for antisera 'A' and arrange the tubes in 1st row from left to right direction in horizontal wooden rack.
- Similarly for titration of antisera 'B' arrange the tubes from 1 to 11th in 2nd row.
- For titration of antisera 'AB' twenty tubes are required (for 'A_1' red cells and 'B' red cells) and arrange them from 1 to 11th in third row and other 11 tubes from 1st to 11th in 4th row.

- Deliver two drops (or 100 µl) of normal saline (0.9%) using standard pasture pipette or 100 µl micropipette from all 2nd (labelled as 1-in-2) to 11th tubes in 1st, 2nd, 3rd and 4th rows (total 40 tubes) leaving the 1st tube in these rows (total 4 tubes labelled as neat).
- Add two drops (or 100 µl) of antisera 'A' (monoclonal) in 1st and 2nd tubes of the 1st row.
- Similarly add two drops (or 100 µl) of antisera 'B' (monoclonal) in 1st and 2nd tubes of the 2nd row.
- Add two drops (or 100 µl) of antisera 'AB' (monoclonal) in 1st and 2nd tubes of the 3rd and 4th rows.
- Mix normal saline and antisera in the second tube of all rows.
- Take two drops (or 100 µl) of diluted antisera 'A' from 2nd tube of 1st row and transfer into 3rd tube. This process is to be done up to 11th tube. Discard two drops (or 100 µl) of diluted antisera from 11th tube or save for further dilution if required.
- Similarly take two drops (or 100 µl) of diluted antisera 'B' from 2nd tube of the 2nd row and transfer into 3rd tube. This process is to be done up to 11th tube. Discard two drops (or 100 µl) of diluted antisera from 11th tube or save for further dilution if required.
- Similarly follow in 3rd and 4th rows, take two drops or 100 µl diluted antisera 'AB' from 2nd tube and transfer into 3rd tube. This process is to be done up to 11th tube. Discard two drops (or 100 µl) of diluted antisera from 11th tube or save for further dilution if required.
- Add one drop (or 50 µl) 5% of corresponding 'A_1' blood group pooled red blood cells suspension in all the tubes from 1st to 11th in 1st row (for antisera 'A' titration).
- Similarly add one drop (or 50 µl) 5% of corresponding 'B' group pooled red blood cells suspension in all the tubes from 1st to 11th in 2nd row (for antisera 'B' titration).
- Add one drop (or 50 µl) 5% of corresponding 'A_1' blood group pooled red blood cells suspension in all the tubes from 1st to 11th in 3rd row (for antisera 'AB' titration).

  Similarly add one drop (or 50 µl) 5% of corresponding 'B' group pooled red blood cells suspension in all the tubes from 1st to 11th in 4th row (for antisera 'AB' titration).
- The 1st tube which has only antisera and corresponding pooled red blood cells suspension is called neat. From 2nd tube to 10th tube according to serial number left to right direction titer ratio is 1-in-2, 1-in-4, 1-in-8, 1-in-16, 1-in-32, 1-in-64, 1-in-128, 1-in-256, 1-in-512, 1-in-1024, respectively.
- Mix gently all tubes from 1st to 4th rows (total 44 tubes) and keep them at room temperature (20–24°C) for 15 minutes (IgM), centrifuge at 1000 rpm for one minute.

  Also follow the instruction of the blood centre SOP.
- **And read the titer:** The titration results should be read from lesser concentration to higher concentration.
- Similarly follow the above-mentioned same titration technique for antisera 'A' where 5% of 'A_2', 'A_1B', and 'A_2B', blood group pooled red blood cells suspension are used.
- Follow the same titration technique for antisera 'B' where 5% of 'A_1B' and 'A_2B' blood group pooled red blood cells suspension are used.

- Follow the same titration technique for antisera 'AB' where 5% of 'A_2', 'A_1B,' and 'A_2B' blood group pooled red blood cells suspension are used.

MASTER DILUTION TECHNIQUE ('A_1','A_2', 'A_1 B' AND 'A_2B') BLOOD GROUP

- Deliver eight drops of normal saline (0.9%) using standard pasture pipette or 400 µl micropipette from all 2nd (labelled as1 in 2) to 11th tubes in 1st row leaving the 1st tube in these rows (as neat).
- Add eight drops (or 400 µl) of antisera 'A' (monoclonal) in 1st and 2nd tube of the 1st row. (1st row for A_1 blood group titration).
- Take two drops (100 ul) of antisera "A" from 1st tube of 1st row to the 1st tubes of 2nd, 3rd and 4th row each.
- Mix normal saline and antisera in the second tube of all 1st to 11th tubes in 1st row.
- Take eight drops (or 400 µl) of diluted antisera 'A' from 2nd tube of 1st row and transfer into 3rd tube. This process is to be done up to 11th tube.
- Take two drops of diluted antisera "A" (100 ul) from 2nd tube of 1st row to 2nd tube of 2nd, 3rd and 4th row. Similarly transfer 100 ul from 3rd to 11th tube of 1st row to their respective tubes of the 2nd, 3rd and 4th rows.
- Add one drop (or 50 µl) 5% of corresponding 'A_1' blood group pooled red blood cells suspension in all the tubes from 1st to 11th in 1st row.
- Similarly add one drop (or 50 µl) 5% of corresponding 'A_2' blood group pooled red blood cells suspension in all the tubes from 1st to 11th in 2nd row.
- Add one drop (or 50 µl) 5% of corresponding 'A_1B' blood group pooled red blood cells suspension in all the tubes from 1st to 11th in 3rd row. Similarly add one drop (or 50 µl) 5% of corresponding 'A_2 B' blood group pooled red blood cells suspension in all the tubes from 1st to 11th in 4th row.
- The 1st tube which has only antisera and corresponding pooled red blood cells suspension is called neat. From 2nd to 10th tubes according to serial number left to right direction titer ratio is 1-in-2, 1-in-4, 1-in-8, 1-in-16, 1-in-32, 1-in-64, 1-in-128, 1-in-256, 1-in-512, 1-in-1024, respectively.
- Mix gently all tubes from 1st to 4th rows (total 44 tubes) and keep them at room temperature (20–24°C) for 45 minutes (IgM), centrifuge at 1000 rpm for one minute. Also follow the instruction of the blood centre SOP.
- **And read the titer:** The titration results should be read from lesser concentration to higher concentration.

Practical Instruction

Titration of antisera 'A' for detection strength of antibodies using 'A_1', 'A_2', 'A_1 B' and 'A_2 B' blood group Rh +Vve or Rh –ve pooled red blood cells suspension, practical preparation of master dilution.

Master dilution titration technique through standard tube method:

- Take 400 µl normal saline 0.9% from 2nd to 11th precipitant tubes except neat.
- Add 400 µl anti-A into 1st and 2nd test tube. Transfer 400 µl diluted antisera from 2nd to 3rd test tube and so on up to 11th test tube and last 400 µl of antisera is either discarded or saved for further testing
- Take three sets of 11 test tubes and labelled as above (Fig. 15.1).

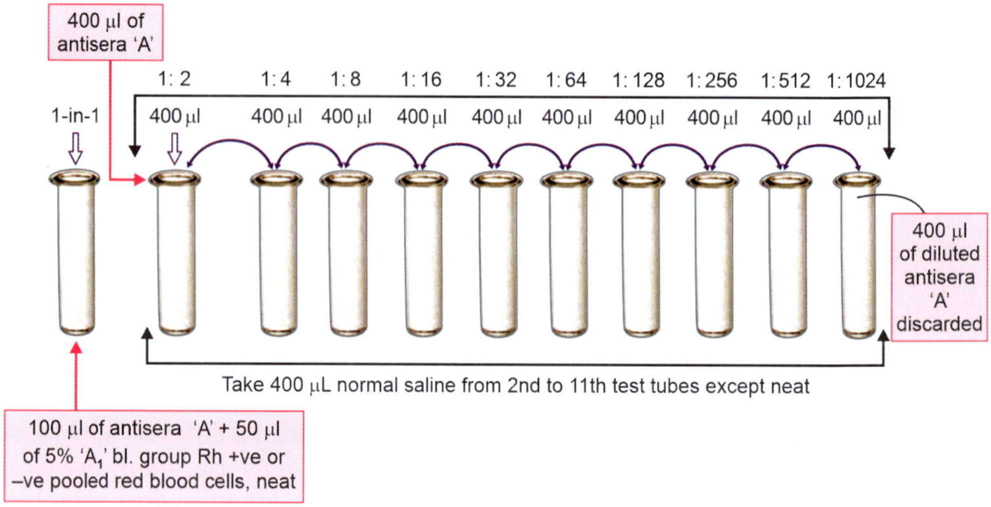

Fig. 15.1: Master dilution technique ('A_1','A_2', 'A_1B' and 'A_2B') blood group

- 1st test tube which has only antisera and corresponding pooled red blood cells suspension is called neat. From 2nd to 11th tubes according to serial number left to right direction titer ratio is 1-in-2, 1-in-4, 1-in-8, 1-in-16, 1-in-32, 1-in-64, 1-in-128, 1-in-256, 1-in-512, 1-in-1024, respectively.
- Transfer 100 µl of diluted antisera 'A' into corresponding tube (1:2 to 1:2 of the 3 sets, 1:32 to 1:32 like this)
- Add A_1, A_2, A_1B and A_2B cells into the respective sets of the test tubes.
- Mix gently all tubes from 1st to 4th row (total 44 tubes) and keep at room temperature (20–24°C) for 45 minutes (IgM), centrifuge at 1000 rpm for one minute.
- **And read the titer:** The titration results should be read from lesser concentration to higher concentration (Tables 15.4a and 15.4b).
- Similarly follow the above-mentioned same titration technique for antisera 'B' where 5% of 'B', 'A_1B' and 'A_2B' group pooled red blood cells suspension are used.
- Follow the same titration technique for antisera 'AB' where 5% of 'A_1', 'A_2', 'A_1B', 'A_2B' and 'B' blood group pooled red blood cells suspension are used.

Table 15.4a: Titration strength for anti-A (monoclonal IgM) reagent with various pooled cells

Type of cells used	*A_1*	*A_2*	*A_2B*	*B*	*O*
Result observation	≥1 : 256	≥1 : 128	≥1 : 64	Negative	Negative
Prozone	Absent	Absent	Absent	Absent	Absent

Table 15.4b: Titration strength for anti-B (monoclonal IgM) reagent

Type of cells used	*B*	*A_1B*	*A_1*	*O*
Result observation	≥1 : 256	≥1 : 128	Negative	Negative
Prozone	Absent	Absent	Absent	Absent

Interpretation

High titer of any antisera indicates the strength of reaction is more in low number of antigens. So, it will prevent any false negative reaction.

TITRATION OF ANTISERA 'D' (IgM) AND 'D' (IgG) MONOCLONAL

Serial dilution technique through standard tube method

Quality Control of Anti-'D' Sera

Rh (D) is most immunogenic and has a higher frequency distribution among all the five varieties of Rh. Quality control of anti-Rh (D) reagents are more complex than ABO reagents because of the great variety of reagents, methods of use and the necessary control procedure.

Each new vial batch titer must be done to know its potency.

Positive and negative controls must be put for validation of results.

Reagents/Apparatus Required

1. Pilot test tubes and 22 precipitin test tubes or standard glass test tubes.
2. Horizontal wooden rack and test tube rack.
3. Micropipette or pasture pipette.
4. Digital bench top centrifuge machine.
5. Digital display incubator.
6. 0.9% of normal saline.
7. Antisera 'D' (IgM or IgM + IgG) and 'D' (IgG) monoclonal.
8. Antihuman globulin (AHG).

- 5% of O Rh +ve red blood cells suspension. 'O' group Rh + ve pooled red blood cells suspension is used for antisera 'D' (IgM and IgG) titer.
- Take 22 precipitin test tubes or standard glass test tubes for antisera 'D' (IgM and IgG, monoclonal) titration.
- Mark on the test tubes from 1 to 11th titration for antisera 'D' (IgM, monoclonal) and arrange the tubes in horizontal wooden rack in 1st row from left to right direction.
- Similarly for antisera 'D' (IgG, monoclonal) titration arrange the tubes from 1st to 11th in 2nd row.
- Deliver two drops (or 100 µl) of normal saline (0.9%) using standard pasture pipette or micropipette from all 2nd (labelled as 1 in 2) to 11th tubes in 1st and 2nd rows (total 20 tubes) leaving the 1st tube in these rows (total 2 tubes labelled as neat).
- Add two drops (or 100 µl) of antisera 'D' (IgM) in 1st and 2nd tubes of the 1st row and antisera 'D'(IgG) in 1st and 2nd tubes of the 2nd row.
- Take two drops (or 100 µl) of diluted antisera 'D'(IgM) from 2nd tube of the 1st row and transfer into 3rd tube. This process is to be done up to 11th tube. Discard two drops (or 100 µl) of diluted antisera from 11th tube or save for further dilution if required.

- Similarly take two drops (or 100 µl) of diluted antisera 'D' (IgG) from 2nd tube of the 2nd row and transfer into 3rd tube. This process is to be done up to 11th tube. Discard two drops (or 100 µl) of diluted antisera from 11th tube or save for further dilution if required.
- Mix normal saline and antisera in 2nd tubes of 1st and 2nd rows.
- Add 5% of Rh D' +Ve 'O' blood group pooled red blood cells suspension in all the tubes from 1st to 11th in 1st and 2nd rows and mix gently all the tubes (Fig. 15.2a). From the 1st to 11th tubes of the 1st row, keep antisera 'D' (IgM) at room temperature (20–24°C) for 15 minutes, centrifuge in 1000 rpm for one minute and read the titer macroscopically and microscopically.
- From the 2nd row antisera 'D' (IgG), incubate all the tubes from the 1st to 11th tubes at 37°C for 45 minutes and wash them three times with normal saline (Fig. 15.2b).
- Decant the supernatant fluid from all the tubes as much as possible.
- Add two drops (or 100 µl) of antihuman globulin (AHG) in all the tubes from 1st to 11th and centrifuge at 1000 rpm for one minute and read the titer immediately macroscopically and microscopically.
- Also follow the instruction of the blood centre SOP.

Practical Instruction

Serial dilution technique through standard tube method:

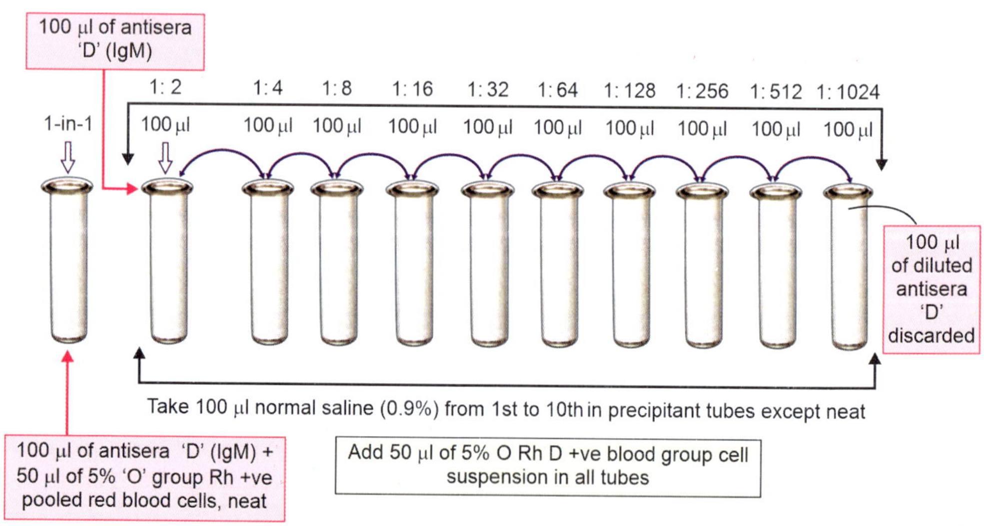

Fig. 15.2a: Titration of antisera 'D' (IgM)

- From 1st row 1st to 11th tubes 'D'(IgM, monoclonal) keep at room temperature (20–24°C) for 15 minutes, centrifuge in 1000 rpm for one minute and read the titer.

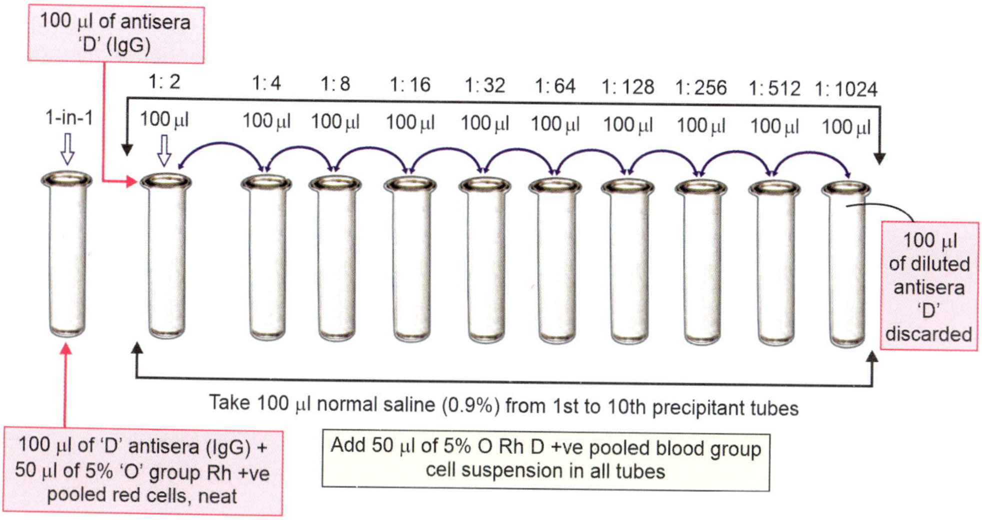

Fig. 15.2b: Titration of antisera 'D' (IgG)

- 1st test tube which has only antisera 'D' and corresponding pooled red blood cells suspension is called neat. From 2nd tube to 11th tube according to serial number left to right direction titer ratio is 1-in-2, 1-in-4, 1-in-8, 1-in-16, 1-in-32, 1-in-64, 1-in-128, 1-in-256, 1-in-512, 1-in-1024, respectively.
- From the 2nd row, incubate antisera 'D' (IgG, monoclonal) in all the tubes from 1st to 11th incubate at 37°C for 45 minutes and wash them three times with normal saline.
- Decant the supernatant fluid from all tubes as much as possible.
- Take two drops (or 100 μl) of antihuman globulin (AHG) in all the tubes from 1st to 11th and centrifuge at 1000 rpm for one minute and read the titer immediately macroscopically and microscopically.
- The titration results should be read from lesser concentration to higher concentration (Table 15.5).

Table 15.5: Titration using anti-D (monoclonal) test result

Type of cells used	*O +Ve*	*Rh negative*
Result observation	1:128	Negative

Interpretation

High titer of anti 'D' antisera can detect 'D' +Ve red blood cells with low amount of antigen expression.

Practical Instruction

Specificity tests for antisera 'A' (monoclonal, IgM) through standard tube technique: Use 2–5% of red blood cells suspension 'A_1', 'A_2' 'B', 'O', 'A_1B' and 'A_2B'groups.

Specificity

- **Specificity check for antisera:** It reacts with corresponding known antigen red cells but does not react with other antigen red cells, e.g. antisera 'A' reacts with 'A_1', 'A_2', 'A_1B' and 'A_2B' blood group antigen but does not react with 'O' and 'B' red blood cells antigen (Fig. 15.3).
- Take twenty different known blood groups and prepare 2–5% of pooled red blood cells suspension.
- Mark on the tubes from 1 to 20 accordingly.
- Take twenty precipitin test tubes or standard glass test tubes and mark on tubes from 1 to 20 accordingly A_1, B, O, A_1 B, A_2 B, B, A_2, A_1, A_1 B, A_1, O, A_1 B, B, A_1, A_2, O, A_1, A_1 B, A_1, B.
- Arrange the tubes on vertical position in the 1st row from left to right direction in horizontal wooden rack.
- Take two drops (or 100 µl) of antisera 'A' in all the tubes from 1st to 20th
- Add one drop (or 50 µl) 2–5% of corresponding 'A_1' blood group red blood cells suspension in the 1st tube, similarly follow 'B' blood group red blood cells suspension in the 2nd tube, 'O' blood group red blood cells suspension in the 3rd tube, 'A_1B' blood group red blood cells suspension in the 4th tube and apply this process up to 20 tubes (prefer 5% of red blood cells suspension for serological tube testing).
- Mix gently antisera and red blood cells suspension in all the tubes from 1st to 20th and incubate them at room temperature (20–24°C) for 45 minutes and centrifuge in 1000 rpm for one minute.
- Observe the result for specificity test.
- Also follow the instruction of the blood centre SOP.
- Result, e.g.: A_1 4+, B–, O–, A_1 B 4+, A_2 B 4+, A_2 3+, etc.
- Similarly apply this process for antisera 'B', 'AB' and lectin 'A1' and follow the steps mentioned above.

Practical Instruction

Add 50 µl 2–5% of different known blood group pooled red blood cells suspension, in each tube.

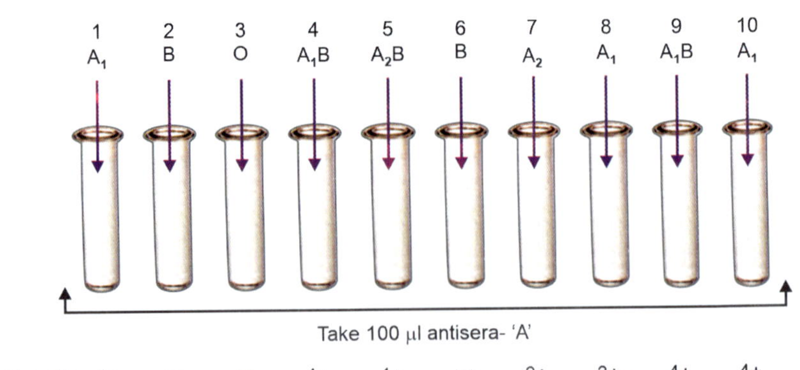

Fig. 15.3: Specificity tests for antisera 'A' (monoclonal, IgM) through standard tube technique

- Mix gently the antisera and red blood cells suspension in all the tubes from 1st to 10th and incubate at room temperature (20–24°C) for 45 minutes and centrifuge at 1000 rpm for one minute.
- Observe the result for specificity test (Fig. 15.3).

Interpretation

Reactive with A cells and no agglutination with B cells.

Avidity

Avidity tests for antisera 'A', 'B' AND 'AB' through glass slide/tile technique:

Speed and strength of agglutination:

- Prepare 50% of 'A_1', 'A_2', 'A_1 B' and 'A_2B' blood group Rh +ve or –ve pooled red blood cells suspension in standard test tubes (12 × 100 mm). It is used for checking avidity of antisera 'A'. Similarly, 'B', 'A_1' 'B', 'A_2 B' group Rh +ve or –ve pooled red blood cells suspension are used for checking avidity of antisera 'B'. 'A_1', 'A_2', 'A_1B', 'A_2B', and 'B' blood group Rh +ve or –ve pooled red cell suspension are used for checking avidity of antisera 'AB'.
- Take a glass slide or tile and put one drop of antisera 'A'. Then put one drop 50% of corresponding 'A_1' blood group pooled red blood cells suspension and rocking it gently at room temperature, and observe the time taken (through stop-watch) for start of agglutination. Similarly apply this procedure for 'A_2', 'A_1B' and 'A_2B' red blood cells for antisera 'B' and 'AB' and follow the abovementioned instruction. Observe agglutination of duration of seconds with the help of stop watch.
- Record the result. Also follow the instruction of blood centre SOP.

Interpretation

The antisera avidity results should meet the standard values in order to meet the quality standards (Table 15.6).

Note: It is the responsibility of the technician in the immunohematology laboratory to ensure that quality-controlled reagents and proper cell concentrations are used for testing and that daily quality control checks and test controls are used with proper documentation. The technician(s) must also ensure that reagents are stored and used as per manufacturer's instruction. This quality control has to be carried out every month and for each new lot.

Table 15.6: Titration requires of antisera 'A', 'B', 'O', 'A_1' 'H' and 'D' (IgM and IgG)

Use of antisera (monoclonal)	*Use of red blood cells*	*Ratio of titer is required (monoclonal)*	*Avidity (monoclonal)*	*Avidity (polyclonol)*
Antisera 'A'	A_1 A_2 A_2B	1-in-256 1-in-128 1-in-64	3–4 seconds 5–6 seconds 5–6 seconds	10–12 seconds 15–18 seconds 15–18 seconds
Antisera 'B'	B A_1B	1-in-256 1-in-128	3–4 seconds 5–6 seconds	10–12 seconds 12–15 seconds
Antisera 'AB'	A_1 B A_2	1-in-256 1-in-256 1-in-128	3–4 seconds 3–4 seconds 5–6 seconds	10–12 seconds 10–12 seconds 15–18 seconds

Contd...

Table 15.6: Titration requires of antisera 'A', 'B', 'O', 'A_1' 'H' and 'D' (IgM and IgG) (*Contd…*)

Use of antisera (monoclonal)	*Use of red blood cells*	*Ratio of titer is required (monoclonal)*	*Avidity (monoclonal)*	*Avidity (polyclonol)*
Lectin extracts				
Antisera 'A_1'	A_1 A_2 O	1-in-32 (A_1), 1-in-16 (A_1B) Negative Negative	15–20 seconds	
Antisera'H'	O A_1 A_2 Oh	1-in-16 1-in-1 1-in-8 Negative	15–20 seconds	
Antisera 'D'				
'D' (IgM)	O	Immediate spin at RT (20–22°C), 1 in 64 to 1 in 128. Incubate at 37°C for 15 minutes. 1:128 to 1:256	5–10 seconds	
'D' (IgM + IgG) monoclonal blend.	O	Immediate spin at RT (20–22°C), 1:32 to 1:64. Incubate at 37°C for 45 minutes. 1:128 to 1:256	10–20 seconds	
'D' (IgG)	O	Incubate at 37°C for 45 minutes. 1:128 to 1:256	15–20 seconds	

Chapter 16

Evaluation of Transfusion Reaction

TRANSFUSION REACTION

Any change in vitals or new onset sign and symptoms during or after completion of transfusion should be taken seriously and to be considered as transfusion reaction until the other causes have been ruled out.

If there is any evidence of significant reactions stop the transfusion but the intravenous line should be kept open with a slow infusion of normal saline. Report to the transfusion service immediately. Different transfusion reactions are depicted in Table 16.1.

Table 16.1: Different types of transfusion reactions

Acute (immediate)
Acute hemolytic transfusion reaction (AHTR)
Febrile nonhemolytic transfusion reaction (FNHTR)
Allergic reaction (urticaria/anaphylaxis)
Transfusion related acute lung injury (TRALI)
Transfusion associated circulatory overload (TACO)
Nonimmune hemolysis (physical/chemical)
Sepsis (bacterial contamination)
Delayed
Delayed hemolytic transfusion reaction (DHTR)
Alloimmunization
Post-transfusion purpura (PTP)
Transfusion associated graft vs host disease (TA-GVHD)
Iron overload
Air embolism

Approach to Transfusion Reaction

- Stop the transfusion
- Maintain intravenous access
- Provide good supportive care
- Contact the transfusion service immediately
- Return implicated blood bag, tags and attached administration set to blood centre
- Check for clerical error (i.e. patient identity and the patient identity on RBC unit).

- Centrifuge post-reaction patient blood sample and examine serum/plasma for hemolysis; if noted, compare with pre-reaction specimen
- Perform DAT; if positive, compare with pre-reaction specimen DAT
- Repeat ABO type of the donor unit, pre- and post-transfusion patient sample
- Repeat antibody screen on the pre- and post-transfusion sample
- Repeat cross-match with the pre- and post-transfusion sample
- If there is evidence of a hemolytic transfusion reaction, additional testing should be performed as needed:
- Laboratory studies for hemoglobinemia and hemoglobinuria (the free hemoglobin causes both plasma and urine to appear red), decreased serum haptoglobin (very sensitive marker of hemolysis) and increased lactate dehydrogenase
- Perform coagulation tests for DIC: PT, APTT, fibrinogen, platelet count
- Maintain good urine output (>1 ml/kg per hour), can use diuretics (furosemide)
- Treat shock and support cardiac and respiratory function

The Transfusion Reaction Workup (*Flowchart 16.1*)

Flowchart 16.1: Showing transfusion reaction workup

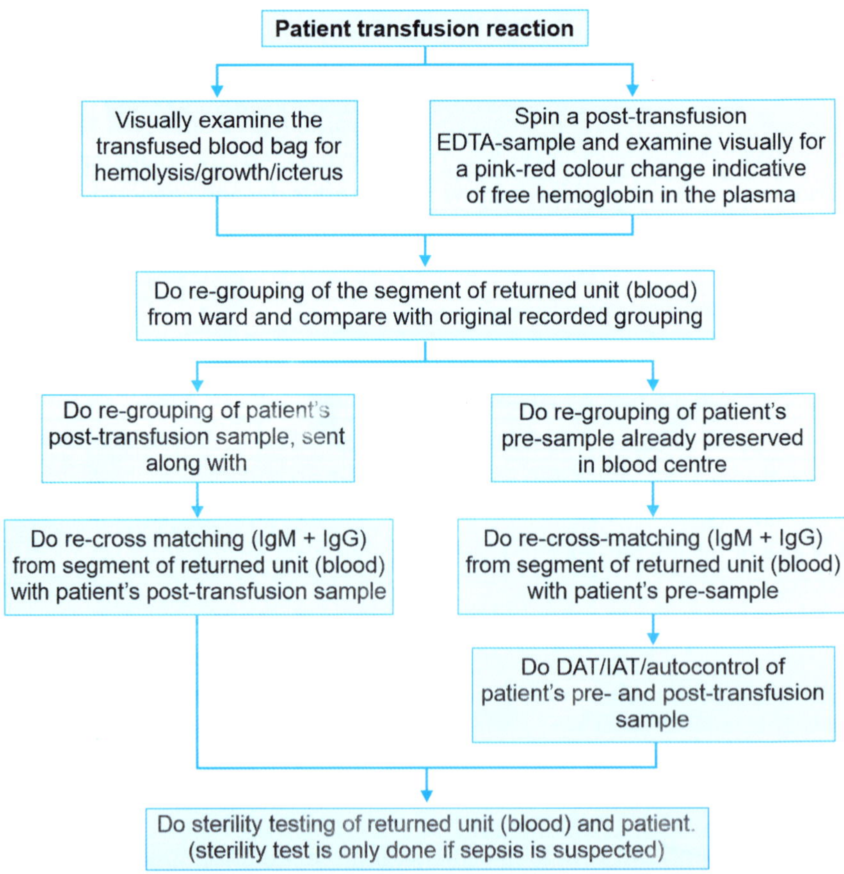

Further Important Investigation

Collect patient urine sample: A red supernatant in the centrifuge urine specimen, positive for hemoglobin. Which for brown as well red urine and check microscopic examination for RBCs (hematuria). Further most important investigation are Serum bilirubin, LDH, blood urea, BUN, serum creatinine and coagulation test like PT, APTT, platelets count, plasma fibrinogen and chest X-ray. All transfusion reaction workup should be carried out under the supervision of transfusion medicine doctor.

Chapter 17

ELISA Technique in Blood Centre

IMMUNOASSAY

A laboratory technique that makes use of the binding between an antigen and its homologous antibody to identify and quantify the specific antigen or antibody in a sample.

Enzyme Linked Immunosorbent Assay (ELISA)

An enzyme linked immunosorbent assay, also called ELISA or EIA.

It is the most commonly used assay and is best on the use of immobilized viral antigen (coated in the wells) which captures anti-HIV antibodies present in the test sample.

This test can be used to determine if you have antibodies related to certain infections conditions. Pre- or post-donation screening of blood donors for transfusion transmissible infection (TTI) ELISA test is the mandatory practice.

These assays may be performed either manually or on automated assay processing systems.

Manufacturers often use the terms first, second, third and fourth generations assay.

The ELISA technique is divided into three types:

1. Competitive ELISA
2. Sandwich ELISA
3. Indirect ELISA

Principle of the HIV Gen^4 Kit

The HIV Gen^4 is a solid phase enzyme linked immunosorbent assay based on the principle of the double antigen/antibody sandwich technique for the detection of the IgM and IgG antibodies against HIV-1 and/or HIV-2 and P^{24} antigen in human serum and plasma.

The HIV Gen^4 is composed by two systems:

1. Solid micro wells pre-coated with:
   a. Recombinant HIV-1 and HIV-2 antigens
   b. Monoclonal anti-P^{24} antibody
2. Liquid conjugates composed of:
   a. Recombinant HIV-1 and HIV-2 antigens conjugate
   b. Monoclonal anti-P^{24} antibody conjugate

In the blood centre commonly sandwich ELISA technique is done for HIV, HBsAg and anti-HCV screening test.

Sandwich ELISA

Principle of the Sandwich ELISA

This is highly specific type of ELISA in which viral antibody in test sample is bound to immobilize antigen (coated in the wells) and then detected by free enzyme-labelled viral antigen.

- Prepare a surface to which a known quantity of capture antibodies is bound.
- Block any non-specific binding sites on the surface.
- Apply the antigen-containing sample to the plate.
- Wash the plate, so that unbound antigen is removed.
- Apply enzyme linked primary antibodies as detection antibodies which also bind specifically to the antigen.
- Wash the plate, so that the unbound antibody-enzyme conjugates are removed.
- Apply a chemical substrate that is converted by the enzyme into a coloured product.
- Measure the absorbency of the plate wells to determine the presence and quantity of antigen.
- ELISA testing material requirement:
  1. Automated ELISA analyzer or ELISA reader (refer to Figs 17.3 and 17.4)
  2. Washer/wash buffer bottle
  3. ELISA test kits
  4. Micropipettes and disposable tips
  5. Timer
  6. Digital display incubator
  7. Digital table top centrifuge machine
  8. Distil/deionized water
  9. Graduated cylinder
  10. Disposable container
  11. Sodium hypochlorite for disposal of waste
  12. Tissue paper
  13. Disposable gloves

Optional (Shaker/Water Bath/Vertex Mixture

ELISA Kit Components

1. **Coated plates:** The 96-well plates are made of polystyrene and coated with either inactivated antigen or antibody. This coating is the binding site for the antibodies or antigens in the sample.
2. Sample diluent/assay buffer
3. Control/standards/calibrator
4. **Conjugate:** ELISA conjugates are enzyme-labelled antibodies or antigens that react specifically to plate-bound sample analytes.

5. **Substrate:** For peroxidase conjugates, the substrate is a mixture of hydrogen peroxide and a chromogen that reacts with the enzyme portion of the conjugate to produce color.
7. **Wash solution:** The wash concentrate is a buffered solution containing detergent used to wash away unbound materials from the microplates.
8. **Stop solution:** The stop solution stops the enzyme-substrate reaction and, thereby, the color development.

Precaution is required before starting the test:

1. Before starting the work read kit instruction carefully.
2. Bring samples at room temperature before testing.
3. Bring all reagents from the freeze 30 minutes prior to testing.
4. Follow manufacturers instruction provided inside the kit for preparation of working wash buffer.
5. Do not use kit/reagent after the expiry date.
6. Standard multi-channel pipette and variable micropipette should be calibrated.
7. Labeling of microplate and strip.

Precaution is required for manually processing system at starting the test

ELISA technology not a childs play, during test run concentration is very much needed. Once the assay has started, complete the procedure without interruption. All the reagents should be dispensed in the centre of the well and the tip of the pipette should not touch the wall of the micro well.

1. Arrange all samples to be tested serially in ascending order in which they are to be tested in test tube rack.
2. Place the microplate in front of the test tube rack.
3. Place the wells strip on the microplate according to the requirement of blank/NC/PC and test samples.
4. Do not pipette by mouth and always use new tips for each sample and reagent.
5. Test samples become free from fibrinogen, hemolysis and lipemic.
6. Add diluents and other reagents into the wells very carefully without bubble formation.
7. Charge or apply reagents/test samples into the wells very carefully at 90° angle by micropipette and avoid any cross-contamination.
8. Mix test sample with respective require reagents into the wells by micropipette very carefully without bubble formation.
9. Mix 10 µl of test serum and controls sample with colorless sample diluent of HCV ELISA test in the wells. Do this process very carefully because 10 µl of test serum and controls sample is very less amount. Some manufacturers have made light color sample diluent in such a way that serum sample and controls samples color changes automatically while mixing. This is technically useful and successful.

10. Do not scratch bottom of the well surface during mixing test samples and require respective reagents by micropipette.
11. Follow strictly manufacturer's instruction provided inside the kit for preparation of working wash buffer, conjugate and other reagents.
12. Follow strictly manufacturer's instruction provided inside the kit for incubation time and washing time of test. Incubation time should not vary by more than ±2 minutes.
13. ELISA plate should be covered with a dark (black) plastic cover during the incubation at 37°C.
14. Before adding redimate substrate into wells for color development (originally is colorless) check if any color is developed in substrate like light blue or white particles then immediately avoid adding otherwise whole procedure will repeat again.
15. Substrate is a highly sensitive reagent. During adding substrate into wells in dark area, do not expose color reagent to light and heat because the color may develop in negative samples and the result shows false positive.
16. After adding substrate reagent if shows a light blue ring or light blue sport at bottom of the well, it means there is cross-contamination and shows the result false reactive and repeat the test.
17. If the sample is reactive and, originally the whole well will develop blue color.
18. Adequate washing of wells is extremely important to avoid any cross contamination of ELISA test in HIV, HBsAg and Anti-HCV.
19. Wash buffer is stable for one month when stored at 2–8°C and follow the manufacturer's instructions.
20. Micro well strip must be taped vigorously. And blotted on blotting or tissue paper to minimize the residual wash buffer.
21. Use a multichannel pipette at manual washing with wash buffer into the wells aspirate completely the contents of all wells by lowering the aspirator tip gently to the bottom of the each well.
22. Use a multichannel pipette at manual washing with wash buffer into the wells do not touch the bottom of the wells surface because there is chance of cross contamination.
23. The dispense height is set to completely fill the well without causing an overflow.
24. Ensure that each row of wells is left to sock time as per the manufacturer's instruction provided inside the kit.
25. Before reporting or discarding the reactive donor's blood bag, always repeat the test in other manufacturer kits for further confirmation.
26. Do not allow the wells to become dry during the assay procedure.
27. Strictly follow the test steps as per manufacturer's instructions provided inside the kit.

Assay Procedure, Steps of the Test

Flowchart 17.1: Steps of ELISA testing for HIV, HBV, HCV (procedures may vary according to the kit in use)

Step	HIV 1-2 Gen^{3} or Gen^{4}/Anti-HCV Gen^{3}	Step	HBsAg Gen^{3}
1st step	Sample diluent/NC/PC and PC^{24}/serum sample	1st step	Sample diluent/NC and PC/ serum sample/conjugate
2nd step	Incubation at 37°C	2nd step	Incubation at 37°C
3rd step	Wash with wash buffer (6 cycles)	3rd step	Wash with wash buffer (6 cycles)
4th step	Conjugate	4th step	Substrate (color reagent)
5th step	Incubation at 37°C	5th step	Incubation at (20–24°C in dark)
6th step	Wash with wash buffer (6 cycles)	6th step	Stop solution
7th step	Substrate (color reagent)	7th step	Reading
8th step	Incubation at (20–24°C in dark)	8th step	Documentation
9th step	Stop solution		
10th step	Reading		
11th step	Documentation		

Reading of the Test

Read the plate at 450 nm (single filter) or using 450 nm and 620/630/650 (double filter).

Follow manufacturers instruction provided inside the kit.

Calculation of results:

Calculate the mean absorbance of the negative controls (Figs 17.1 and 17.2).

> ***Example:***
> Mean negative control = (Abs B1 + Abs C1 + Abs D1) ÷ 3
> Cut-off value = Mean NC + Cut-off factor
> Cut-off factor is already provided in individual kit.
> If negative control absorbance results show 0.072 + 0.021 + 0.033 = 0.126 ÷ 3 = 0.042, then add mean value and cut-off factor
> If cut-off factor is 0.1
> 0.1 + 0.042 = 0.142 = Cut-off value

Grey zone area:

If result of test sample is within 10% of cut-off value then repeat the test for further confirmation.

1. If the cut-off value is 0.142 and the test value is between 0.128 and 0.142, then this value will be considered as grey zone (0.142 ÷ 10 = 0.0142) 0.142–0.0142 = 0.1278 (test value).

TEST VALUE ABOVE CUT-OFF VALUE IS REACTIVE AND BELOW CUT-OFF VALUE IS NON-REACTIVE

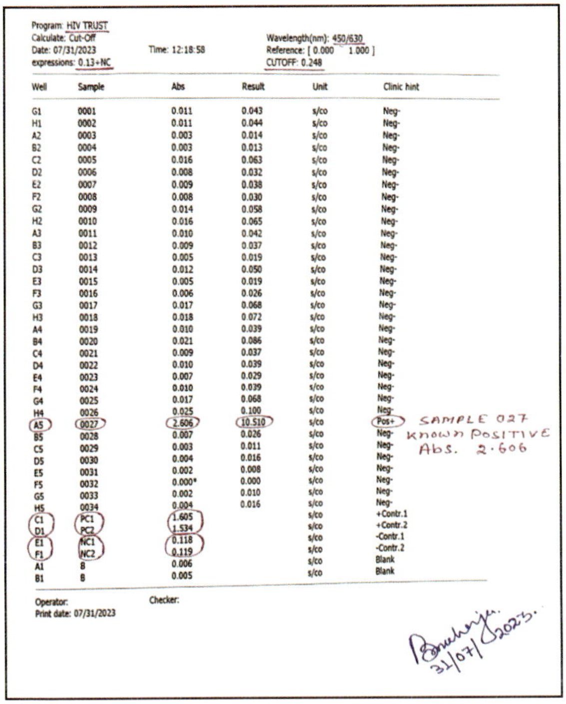

Program: HIV TRUST
Calculate: Cut-Off
Date: 07/31/2023 Time: 12:18:58
expressions: 0.13+NC
Wavelength(nm): 450/630
Reference: [0.000 1.000]
CUTOFF: 0.248

Well	Sample	Abs	Result	Unit	Clinic hint
G1	0001	0.011	0.043	s/co	Neg-
H1	0002	0.011	0.044	s/co	Neg-
A2	0003	0.003	0.014	s/co	Neg-
B2	0004	0.003	0.013	s/co	Neg-
C2	0005	0.016	0.063	s/co	Neg-
D2	0006	0.008	0.032	s/co	Neg-
E2	0007	0.009	0.038	s/co	Neg-
F2	0008	0.008	0.030	s/co	Neg-
G2	0009	0.014	0.058	s/co	Neg-
H2	0010	0.016	0.065	s/co	Neg-
A3	0011	0.010	0.042	s/co	Neg-
B3	0012	0.009	0.037	s/co	Neg-
C3	0013	0.005	0.019	s/co	Neg-
D3	0014	0.012	0.050	s/co	Neg-
E3	0015	0.005	0.019	s/co	Neg-
F3	0016	0.006	0.026	s/co	Neg-
G3	0017	0.017	0.068	s/co	Neg-
H3	0018	0.018	0.072	s/co	Neg-
A4	0019	0.010	0.039	s/co	Neg-
B4	0020	0.021	0.086	s/co	Neg-
C4	0021	0.009	0.037	s/co	Neg-
D4	0022	0.010	0.039	s/co	Neg-
E4	0023	0.007	0.029	s/co	Neg-
F4	0024	0.010	0.039	s/co	Neg-
G4	0025	0.017	0.068	s/co	Neg-
H4	0026	0.025	0.100	s/co	Neg-
A5	0027	2.606	10.510	s/co	Pos+
B5	0028	0.007	0.026	s/co	Neg-
C5	0029	0.003	0.011	s/co	Neg-
D5	0030	0.004	0.016	s/co	Neg-
E5	0031	0.002	0.008	s/co	Neg-
F5	0032	0.000*	0.000	s/co	Neg-
G5	0033	0.002	0.010	s/co	Neg-
H5	0034	0.004	0.016	s/co	Neg-
C1	PC1	1.605		s/co	+Contr.1
D1	PC2	1.534		s/co	+Contr.2
E1	NC1	0.118		s/co	-Contr.1
F1	NC2	0.119		s/co	-Contr.2
A1	B	0.006		s/co	Blank
B1	B	0.005		s/co	Blank

SAMPLE 027 KNOWN POSITIVE Abs. 2.606

Operator: Checker:
Print date: 07/31/2023

31/07/2023.

Fig. 17.1: HIV, ELISA test (Gen[3]) test report

Note: In this ELISA report, negative control (NC) is tested in well E1 and F1 and positive control (PC) in well C1 and D1 and a known positive control in well A1. The cut off value is 0.248. The absorbance (Abs) value for E1 and F1 is <0.248 and Abs value for C1, D1 and A1 (known positive control) is >0.248. Hence the test result is valid.

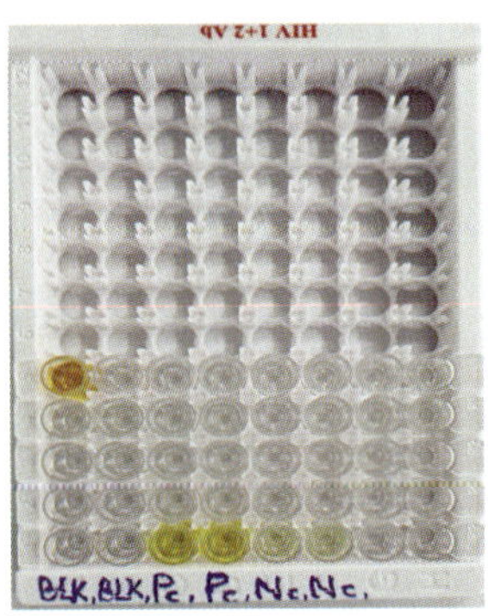

Fig. 17.2: ELISA microplate

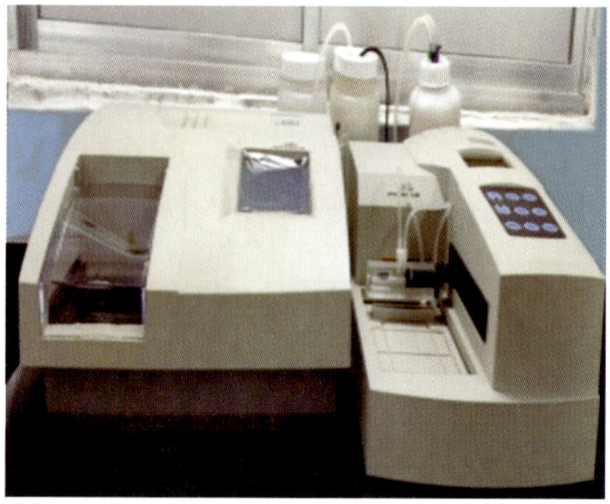

Fig. 17.3: ELISA reader and washer

AUTOMATED ELISA PROCESSOR

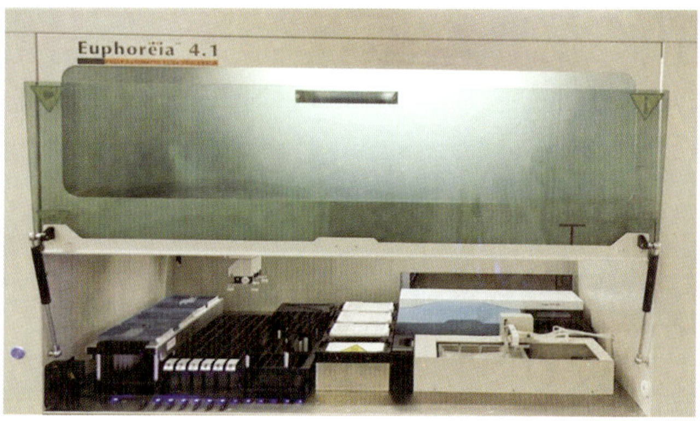

Fig. 17.4: Automated ELISA processor

KEY FEATURES

Following key features are available in automated ELISA processor.

1. High speed robotic arm.
2. Robotic washer.
3. Robotic reader.
4. Reagent container and tips racks.
5. Sample tubes and control vials rails (channels).
6. Flexible modular platform.
7. Incubator.
8. Software.

OPERATING PROTOCOL FOR AUTOMATED ELISA PROCESSOR

- Prepare wash buffer according to manufacturer's instruction provided inside the kit and fill in the appropriate number in wash buffer bottle.

- Fill distilled water sufficient in the appropriate number in wash bottle.
- Switch on the instrument followed by the CPU of the machine.
- Open the ELISA processing software from desktop.
- Open the "Maintenance" icon from "Home" window.
- Keep wash cycle "Prime Run" and click on "Start" 4 times before the test run and complete the test run.
  - (Properly observe the uniform flow of liquid from dispensing needles and aspiration needles of the wash manifold).
- Open "Start running" option for preparing the work list.
- Create the work list from "New batch" option.
- Open the "Running gante" window, check (√) on "Simular running" and click on "Start".
- Select the tip rack and reagent position.
- Once software shows "Running is completed" click on "Yes".
- Properly place the sample tubes and control vials into the respective rails (channels hole).
- From "Workflow" window observe the required volume of each reagent and number of micro wells for each test. Prepare the working reagent and keep all reagents in appropriate position.
- Place the respective microplate with required micro well strip into appropriate position.
- Load the sufficient number of tips for samples and reagents in the tips rack.
- Finally check the number of tips, reagent container, microplate and microplate lid properly in respective position.
- Open the "Running gante" window, uncheck (√) the "Simular running" and click on "Start". Test process will be completed according to the time schedule provided in manufacturer's instruction written inside the kit
- Open "Test result" window to see the plate result.
- "Lock" the result for taking the print out.
- Open the "Maintenance" icon from "Home" window.
- Select the distilled water bottle and "Wash cycle" 4 times click on "Start".
- Switch Off the instrument followed by shut-down the CPU.

Note: Steps and procedures of "ELISA processor" may differ from machine to machine (automated) and it should follow the manufacturer's manual instruction and blood centre SOP.

Chapter 18

Hemoglobin Determination by Portable HemoCue System and $CuSO_4$ Method

HEMOGLOBIN DETERMINATION BY HEMOCUE

Principle

The HemoCue Hb (Hemoglobin) testing system is used for the quantitative determination of hemoglobin and calculated hematocrit (HCT) in finger prick single drop of whole blood or venous human whole blood. The system consists of the analyser and specially cuvettes containing dried reagents. The hemoglobin measurement takes place in the analyser and is factory calibrated against the hemoglobin cyanide (HiCN) method. Sodium deoxycholate hemolyses the erythrocytes and hemoglobin is released. Sodium nitrite converts hemoglobin to methaemoglobin which, together with sodium azide gives azide methaemoglobin.

Hemoglobin determination by HemoCue system (Figs 18.1 to 18.3) is the best and accurate method. These are portable and simple to use for donor measuring hemoglobin estimation and the detailed steps to measure Hb is depicted in Flowchart 18.1).

Advantages of HemoCue System

- Accuracy of hemoglobin test result.
- Haemoglobin testing system provides results in less than 15 seconds.
- Easy to use and can be carried from blood centre to blood donation camp centre.
- Quick quantitative result.
- Automatically checks the intensity of light and operation of photo cells.
- No blood dispensing, pippetting or mixing of blood with the reagent.
- Touch display, bar-code, scanner, and automatic transfer of results makes treating doctors.

Hemoglobin results	*Interpretation*
Hemoglobin <12.5 gm/dL	Defer
Hemoglobin >12.5 gm/dL	Accept

Flowchart 18.1: Hemoglobin ditermination by HemoCue system

The preferred site for collection of a capillary blood sample is from the middle or ring finger of children or adults sample at the side of the fingertip for best blood flow and comfort

↓

Press lightly towards fingertip and puncture using a lancet

↓

Wipe away the first and second drop with a clean, dry gauze or lint free tissue press lightly towards fingertip until another drop of appears (do not use cotton balls since cotton fibers will interfere with the test)

↓

Collect the third drop of blood for analysis

↓

When the blood drop is large enough, fill the microcuvette completely in one step. (Do not refill) avoid touching the microcuvette to the skin

↓

After feeling the single drop of blood into the microcuvette, remove the extrablood by using lint-free tissue paper

↓

Insert the microcuvette into the HemoCue system

↓

Follow section measurement procedure to perform measurement whilst measuring will be displayed

↓

The result is displayed as long as the cuvette holder is in measuring Note down the value on the screen position

↓

Discard the microcuvette after measurement microcuvettes are for single use only

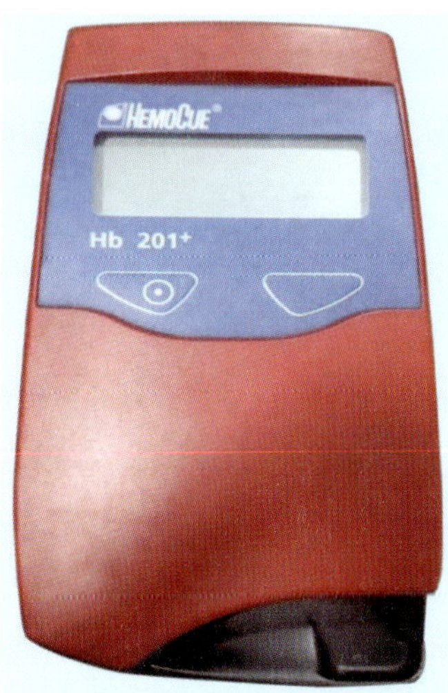

Fig. 18.1: HemoCue portable system

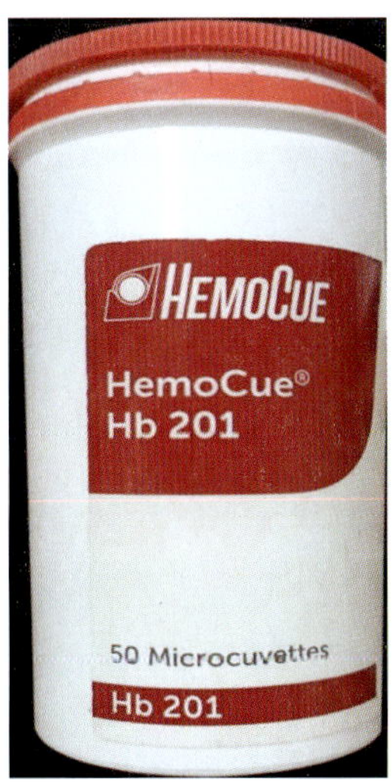

Fig. 18.2: Microcuvette bottle

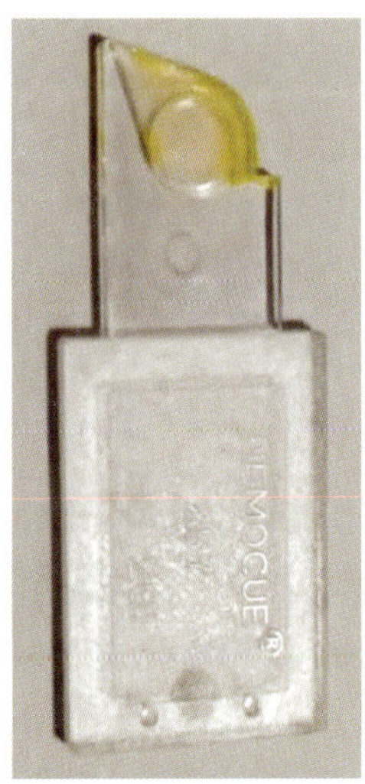

Fig. 18.3: Microcuvette

ESTIMATION OF HEMOGLOBIN BY COPPER SULPHATE ($CuSO_4$) SOLUTION

Principle

This method is based on specific gravity. This is not a quantitative test; it is a semi-quantitative test which shows only whether the hemoglobin is below or above acceptable limits. A drop of blood dropped into $CuSO_4$ of specific gravity 1.053 becomes encased in a sac of copper proteinate, which prevents any change in specific gravity for about 15 seconds.

If the hemoglobin is equal to or more than 12.5 gm/dl the drop will sink within 15 seconds and the donor is accepted.

Reagents/Apparatus Required

1. Copper sulphate crystals ($CuSO_4$).
2. Measuring cylinder 1000 ml and 100 ml.
3. Hydrometer.
4. Conical flask 1000 ml, 500 ml and 250 ml as per requirement.
5. Conical funnel.
6. Glass bottle container with capped.
7. Digital wing machine.
8. Approx 30 ml of capacity glass coplin container (jar).
9. Distil water

Preparation of $CuSO_4$ stock solution (specific gravity 1.100)

Weight exactly 159.6 gm of dry and pure $CuSO_4$ crystals into a conical flask and dissolve in distil water. And make final volume up to 1000 ml. Specific gravity of the stock solution made is 1.100. Cap the conical flask and mix well to ensure that the copper sulphate has dissolved.

Precaution: Copper sulphate crystals are dissolved in distil water very slowly. During preparation add distil water in $CuSO_4$ slowly-slowly and at that time shake continuously conical flask by hand. This process is to be continued till dissolve completely $CuSO_4$ in distil water.

Steps of the Hb Estimation Test

Preparation of $CuSO_4$ working solution for hemoglobin estimation (specific gravity 1.053).

Measure out 520 ml of stock solution prepared into a conical flask and dilute with distil water and make final volume up to 1000 ml (520 ml prepared $CuSO_4$ + 480 ml distil water).

Or add 52 ml of prepared stock solution to 48 ml of distil water to make 100 ml of working solution. Check the specific gravity (of 1.053) by hydrometer.

It should be stored in a tightly capped container to prevent evaporation. The solution should be kept at room temperature before it is used.

Steps of the Hemoglobin Estimation Test by Copper Sulphate Method

1. Dispense a sufficient amount (approx 30 ml) of copper sulphate working solution in a clean, dry glass coplin container (jar) is used for determining hemoglobin.
2. The jar is kept covered with a lid when not in use.

3. Clean the site of fingertip puncture thoroughly with a spirit swab and allowed it to dry.
4. Finger tip puncture with sterile disposable lancet or needle.
5. The first drop of blood is wiped and next drop of blood is allowed to fall gently at about 1 cm above the copper sulphate solution.
6. Observe for more than 15 seconds.
7. Dispose of the disposable needles or lancet and blood-contaminated cotton/gauze in an appropriate container for disposal. (Lancets or needles are disposed off in a container with 1% sodium hypochlorite solution.)

Interpretation

- If the drop of blood has a higher specific gravity (Hb% >12.5 gm), it will sink within 15 seconds to the bottom of the solution.
- If Hb% is <12.5 gm, i.e. specific gravity <1.053 the blood drop will remain suspended or floats within 15 seconds to the top of the solution.
- If the drop sinks slowly, hesitates and then goes to the bottom of the jar, confirm the hemoglobin of this donor.
- If the $CuSO_4$ test could not confirm the status of the donor, repeat hemoglobin by Sahlis/Drabkin's/automated cell counter.
- Change the working solution daily or after 25 tests.

Hemoglobin concentration and interpretation

Results	*Hemoglobin concentration*	*Interpretation*
Blood drop floats	Hemoglobin <12.5 gm/dL	Defer
Blood drop sinks	Hemoglobin >12.5 gm/dL	Accept

FURTHER READING

1. Cohn CS, Delaney M, Johnson ST, Katz LM, Schwartz JY, editors. AABB Technical Manual. 21st ed. AABB Press; 2023.
2. Dixon, LA, and Hemphill, RR (2016). Acquired hemolytic anemia. Tintinalli's emergency medicine: A comprehensive study guide. 8th ed. Oxford: McGraw-Hill.
3. Ewald, DR, and Sumner, SC (2016). Blood type biochemistry and human disease. Wiley Interdisciplinary Reviews: Systems Biology and Medicine, 8(6), 517–35.
4. Harmening, DM (2018). Modern blood banking and transfusion practices. FA Davis.
5. Judd, WJ (1999). Modern approaches to pretransfusion testing. Immunohematology, 15(1), 41–52.
6. Makroo, RN. (2011). Transfusion medicine. Apollo Medicine, 8(4), 319.
7. Mollison, PL (2014). Engelfriet CP, Contreras M Blood Transfusion in Clinical Medicine-12th Ed.-Blackwell Scientific Publications-Oxford.
8. Petz, LD, and Garratty, G (1980). Acquired immune hemolytic anemias. Newyork: Curchill Livingstone.
9. Reference: www. Ortho-clinical diagnostics.
10. Rudmann, SV (2005). Textbook of blood banking and transfusion medicine. Elsevier Health Sciences.
11. Simon, TL, McCullough, J, Snyder, EL, Solheim, BG, and Strauss, RG (Eds). (2022). Rossi's principles of transfusion medicine. John Wiley and Sons, Incorporated.
12. Standards for Blood Banks and Blood Transfusion Services (NACO). 2007.
13. Training Module for Blood Centre, NBTC, NACO, 2015.
14. Transfusion Medicine Technical Manual, DGHS, 3rd Edition 2022.
15. www.tulipgroup.com

PART

II

Advance Techniques of Blood Components Preparation

Chapter 1

Blood Components and their Functions

Blood components are various parts of blood like red blood cells (RBCs), platelets, granulocytes, and plasma. The components can be separated from one another by centrifugation because of their different specific gravities, using different centrifugal forces, different times, and different temperature according to the need.

1. **Cellular components:** RBCs or packed red blood cells, platelets concentrate, granulocytes.
2. **Non-cellular plasma components:** Fresh frozen plasma, cryoprecipitate, and cryo-poor plasma.

FUNCTIONS OF BLOOD COMPONENTS

- **RBC:** It supplies oxygen to different parts of the body and carries carbon dioxide and other waste products.
- **Platelets:** Platelets are produced in the bone marrow. The function of platelets is to prevent bleeding (important for blood clotting).
- **WBC:** It fights/prevents infections of diseases. White blood cells (WBCs) producing antibodies to develop immunity against infections.

Human blood consists of 55% plasma, 45% RBC, 0.1% WBC and 0.17% platelets	In plasma, available stable coagulation factors are fibrinogen, FVII, FX, FXI, FXIII, etc. and unstable (labile) factors are FV and FVIII

- **Plasma:** It is the liquid part of blood, composed of about 92% water, 7% vital proteins such as albumin, gamma globulin, anti-hemophilic factor, and other clotting factors, and 1% mineral salts, sugars, fats, hormones and vitamins.

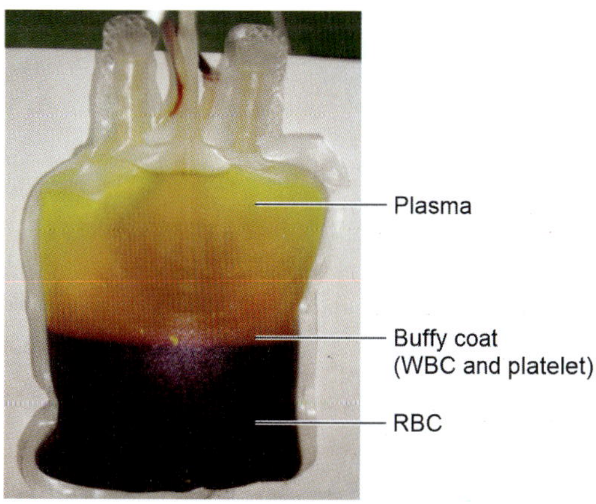

Fig. 1.1: Layers of whole blood after centrifugation

Chapter 2

Introduction to Blood Components

The separation of blood components from whole blood is very useful for modern medical practice. In developing countries, there is large gap between the demand and supply of blood units. Because of the poor awareness of blood donations among the eligible blood donors, there is shortage of voluntary blood donation in most part of the world. Hence, blood component preparation is essential to reduce the demand-supply gap. From one unit of whole blood, one or more blood components like packed red cells (PRC), platelet concentrate (random donor platelet: RDP), fresh frozen plasma (FFP) and cryoprecipitate are prepared. The advantage lies in the fact that the components prepared from one unit of whole blood can now be utilized for more than one patient, the only appropriate component of the blood being used up by the patients as per their needs (Flowchart 2.1).

Flowchart 2.1: Targeted component therapy

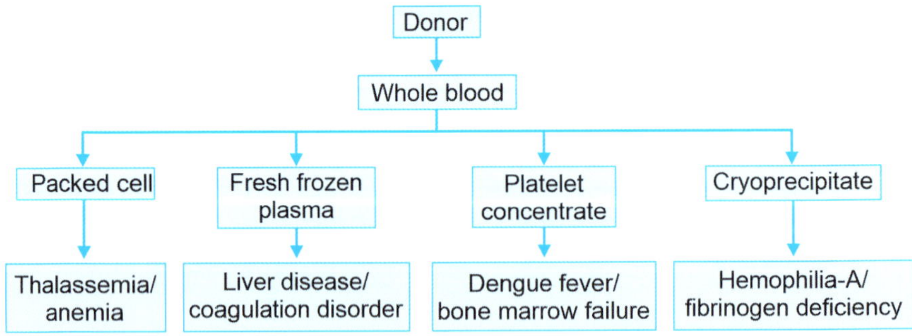

Excess plasma available in a unit of whole blood is not beneficial for the treatment of anemia; instead, it causes volume overload and cardiac, and respiratory complications. So, the plasma is separated from whole blood to prepare the PRC which will treat anemia. Plasma, the liquid portion of the blood, contains albumin, globulin, fibrinogen, and other coagulation factors. Hence, FFP is utilized to treat coagulation disorders. Cryoprecipitate that is prepared from fresh frozen plasma is rich in factor VIII, vWF, and fibrinogen and considered to treat factor-deficient disorders like afibrinogenemia/ hypofibrinogenemia, vWD. Thus, one important component which is not necessary for one patient, may be conserved for the other patients. **Thus, a single unit of whole blood can save four lives.** The targeted component therapy can be achieved by aphaeresis technique also, where an apheresis machine collects a single or multicomponent.

The usage of fresh whole blood refrigerated (2–6°C) has no significance in the practical field apart from acute hemorrhagic conditions like accidental trauma requiring massive transfusion, PPH (postpartum hemorrhage), and double volume exchange transfusion (DVET) for hyperbilirubinemia in a newborn baby. A PRC compatible with both mother and baby is suspended in AB plasma and utilized for DVET.

Chapter 3

Modifications of Blood Components and their Advantages

Modifications of blood components refer to various processes used to alter blood products for specific medical needs, ensuring safety and efficacy in transfusions and other treatments. Here are some common modifications:

1. Leukoreduction

- **Purpose:** Removes white blood cells (leukocytes) from blood products.
- **Reason:** Reduces the risk of febrile non-hemolytic transfusion reactions (FNHTR), transmission of leukocyte-associated viruses, and alloimmunization.
- **Indication:**
  - Multitransfused patients like thalassemia, sickle cell disease, and oncology patients with a risk of alloimmunization.
  - Patients with a previous history of FNHTR
  - Cytomegalovirus-negative patient requiring transfusion or transplant.

2. Irradiation

- **Purpose:** Exposes cellular blood components to gamma rays or X-rays.
- **Reason:** Prevents transfusion-associated graft-versus-host disease (TA-GVHD) by inactivating T-lymphocytes in the blood.
- **Indications:**
  - Transplant patients
  - Immunocompromised patients
  - Intrauterine transfusion
  - Rare blood group from first-degree relatives

3. Washing

- **Purpose:** Removes plasma proteins, electrolytes, and other substances from red blood cells or platelets.
- **Reason:** Reduces allergic reactions in patients sensitive to plasma proteins and prevents hyperkalemia in neonates.
- **Indications:**
  - Patients who have a history of severe allergic reactions, including anaphylaxis, to plasma proteins.
  - Patients with IgA deficiency who have developed anti-IgA antibodies

- In neonates, to reduce potassium in blood components
- Patients with PNH, a rare blood disorder where washing reduces the risk of complement-mediated hemolysis
- Patients with renal failure, infants, or others at risk for hyperkalemia
- Patients who have experienced FNHTRs during previous transfusions.

4. Pooled Plasma or Platelet

- **Purpose:** Same as that of FFP (bleeding patients, massive transfusion) or RDP.
- **Reason:**
  - Pooled plasma—ensure a consistent product with a broader range of clotting factors. Pooling neutralises or dilutes the HLA antibodies.
  - Pooled platelet—platelets from multiple donors are pooled to achieve a sufficient therapeutic dose for transfusion.
- **Indications:**
  - Pooled plasma:
    - Coagulation factor deficiency, massive transfusion, liver disease, TTP
    - Prevents TRALI
  - Pooled platelet:
    - Same as RDP—bleeding due to thrombocytopenia, or platelet dysfunction.

5. Pathogen Reduction

- **Purpose:** Reduces the risk of transfusion-transmitted infections by inactivating pathogens.
- **Reason:** Increases safety by lowering the risk of viral, bacterial, and parasitic infections.

6. Volume Reduction

- **Purpose:** Removes a portion of the plasma or additive solution to concentrate the cellular components.
- **Reason:** Useful for patients who need a small volume of blood components, such as neonates or those with volume overload concerns.

7. Cryopreservation

- **Purpose:** Freezes blood products, particularly rare blood types or autologous units, for long-term storage.
- **Reason:** Allows blood to be stored for years, making it available when needed, especially in cases of rare blood types.

8. Deglycerolization

- **Purpose:** Removes glycerol from cryopreserved red blood cells after thawing.
- **Reason:** Ensures the cells are safe for transfusion after thawing, typically done before transfusion.

9. Platelet Additive Solutions (PAS)

- **Purpose:** Suspends platelets in a specially formulated solution instead of plasma.
- **Reason:** Reduces allergic reactions and improves platelet storage conditions.

These modifications are vital in modern transfusion medicine, enhancing the safety and effectiveness of blood products tailored to patient needs.

Chapter 4

Blood Donor Selection and Blood Collection

Safe blood is essential for each patient and its availability is possible by collecting blood from safe donor, screening the donor effectively through proper donor questionnaires and advanced testing methods for transfusion transmitted infections. Blood donor selection is the most important and preliminary step of transfusion service. Blood must be collected from healthy, non-remunerated and safe donors to avoid any unwanted effects on the recipient.

A blood donor is selected based on the selection criteria described below.

General Selection Criteria

- A safe donor means he is in good health, mentally alert and physically fit.
- He/she shall not be inmates of jail or any other confinement.
- Differently abled or donor with communication and sight difficulties can donate blood provided that clear and confidential communication can be established and he/she fully understands the donation process and gives a valid consent.
- A donor can donate from minimum age of 18 years to 65 years, but cannot donate after 60 years of age if not donated previously. For apheresis donation also age limit is from 18 to 60 years.
- Donation interval should be once in three months (90 days) for males and four months (120 days) for females for whole blood donation. For apheresis, at least 48 hours interval after platelet/plasma—apheresis shall be kept (not more than 2 times a week, limited to 24 in one year).
- After whole blood donation a plateletpheresis donor shall not be accepted before 28 days. Apheresis platelet donor shall not be accepted for whole blood donation before 28 days from the last platelet donation provided reinfusion of red cell was complete in the last plateletpheresis donation. If the reinfusion of red cells was not complete then the donor shall not be accepted within 90 days.
- A donor shall not donate any type of donation within 12 months after a bone marrow harvest, within 6 months after a peripheral stem cell harvest.
- The donor should neither be in empty stomach nor with heavy meal prior to blood donation.
- Donor shall not have consumed alcohol and show signs of intoxication before the blood donation. The donor shall not be a person having regular heavy alcohol intake.

- The donor who works as air crew member, long distance vehicle driver, either above sea level or below sea level or in emergency services or where strenuous work is required, shall not donate blood at least 24 hours prior to their next duty shift. The donor shall not be a night shift worker without adequate sleep.
- The donor shall not be a person considered—at risk for HIV, hepatitis B or C infections (transgender, men who have sex with men, female sex workers, injecting drug users, persons with multiple sexual partners or any other high-risk as determined by the medical officer deciding fitness to donate blood).
- The donor shall not be a person with history of residence or travel in a geographical area which is endemic for diseases that can be transmitted by blood transfusion and for which screening is not mandated or there is no guidance in India.
- If a non-resident of India wants to donate blood, he/she should have stayed in India for three years continuously.

Physical and Medical Selection Criteria

- Minimum weight should be >45 kg to collect 350 ml and >55 kg to collect 450 ml, and for apheresis donation >50 kg.
- Height is measured for apheresis donor.
- Blood pressure, pulse, respiratory rate and temperature of the donor should be normal (systolic 100–140 mm Hg and diastolic 60–90 mmHg, pulse—60–100/min). Donors with antihypertensive medication can donate if there is no change in medication or its dose for the last 28 days and BP is normal during this period.
- A donor should have minimum Hb 12.5 gm/dl.
- For platelet donors, platelet count should be >1.5 lakh/cmm and the peripheral venous access should be prominent.
- Female donor should be deferred during the period of menstruation or breastfeeding.
- A donor with diabetes mellitus well controlled by diet or oral hypoglycemic medication, with no history of orthostatic hypotension and no evidence of infection, neuropathy or vascular disease (in particular peripheral ulceration) can be accepted for donation. The deferral criterias for different medical and surgical causes are depicted in Table 4.1.
- Skin at the phlebotomy site should be free from infections. Needle prick injuries should be looked for among the IV drug users or professional blood donors.

Temporary and Permanent Deferral Criteria

Table 4.1: Enumerates the temporary deferral criteria for a donor

Deferral reason	*Deferral period*
Ketoconazole, antihelminthic drugs including mebendazole	7 days after last dose
Fever, flu	15 days after recovery
Antibiotics, ticlopidine, clopidogrel, piroxicam, dipyridamole	2 weeks after last dose
Non live vaccines and toxoid: Typhoid, cholera, papillomavirus, influenza, meningococcal, pertussis, pneumococcal, polio injectable, diphtheria, tetanus, plague)	2 weeks
Live attenuated vaccines: Polio oral, measles (rubella), mumps, yellow fever, japanese encephalitis, influenza, typhoid, cholera, hepatitis A	28 days

(Contd...)

Table 4.1: Enumerates the temporary deferral criteria for a donor (*Contd...*)	
Deferral reason	*Deferral period*
Anti-tetanus serum, anti-venom serum, anti-diphtheria serum, and anti-gas gangrene serum	28 days
Chickenpox, measles, mumps	2 weeks after recovery
Finasteride used to treat benign prostatic hyperplasia	1 month after the last dose
Etretinate, acitretin or isotretinoin	1 month from last dose
Radioactive contrast material	8 weeks
History of malaria	3 months (endemic)
Zika virus/west nile virus	4 months after recovery
Dutasteride used to treat benign prostatatic hyperplasia	6 months from last dose
Dengue, chikungunya	6 months after recovery
Abortion	6 months
Minor surgery	6 months
Typhoid	12 months
Gamma globulin/HBV immunoglobulin	12 months
Rabies vaccination	12 months
Hepatitis in family or close contact	12 months
Tattoo, ear puncture	12 months
History of blood transfusion	12 months
Major surgery	12 months
Jaundice	12 months
Tuberculosis	2 years after complete treatment

Defer the Donor Permanently if Suffering from any of the Following Diseases

- Cancer
- Heart disease
- Abnormal bleeding tendencies
- Diabetes—on insulin
- Hepatitis B and C infections
- Chronic nephritis
- Chronic liver disease
- Asthma on steroid
- Epilepsy
- Leprosy
- Schizophrenia
- Endocrine disorders
- Kala-azar
- Cerebrovascular diseases
- Recipients of growth hormones or factor VIII conc, bleeding disorder, polycythemia vera, hemoglobinopathies.

- Syphilis, gonorrhea, known or at risk of HIV.
- Autoimmune disorder.

Consent from the donor:

- Prior to donation, inform the donor regarding the process of blood donation, risk associated, information regarding transfusion-transmitted infection (TTI) screening, and component preparation.
- Ask the donor if he/she wants to be notified of the abnormal results of TTI screening.
- Obtain written consent on the blood donor registration card (for donors who cannot sign, a thumb impression may be obtained).
- Inform regarding the release of surplus plasma to the fractionation center and take the consent for the same.

Donor registration:

- If the donor meets the selection criteria, accept the donor for blood donation.
- Assign a specific donor registration number.
- Enter the number on the donor's registration form, donor register and blood bag.
- Accompany the donor for phlebotomy or request to wait if the donor couch is not available.

Note: For optimum quality component preparation whole blood required is 450 ml because optimum platelets yields and adequate plasma volume are available.

General awareness for donors:

Blood donation is a great contribution to our society. It is a safe procedure. A healthy and regular voluntary donor is an ideal candidate to donate blood as the risk of transfusion-transmitted infections is less. Blood donation is carried out under the supervision of a doctor (transfusion medicine or trained doctor), trained skilled technicians, and nurse. Our mission is to collect safe blood from a regular donor.

Some important recommendations for the donor before and during donation of blood.

1. Before donating, fill up a donor questionnaire form and write answers very carefully.
2. If you have come from a long drive, take rest for at least 30 minutes and then donate blood.
3. Do not give blood on an empty stomach.
4. Eat a well-balanced diet including plenty of fluids before blood donation.
5. Do not open shoes before sitting on donor couch/chair. If you tie up shoe lace after donation, blood may come out from bleeding point and may increase the risk of vasovagal.
6. A loose dress should be preferred at the time of donating blood.
7. No pressure creating external device/thread should be in forearm of the donor from which blood is being drawn.
8. During blood donation, be relax, listen to music and talk to other donors or technical staff.

9. Donor must be kept under strict observation during and after donation.
10. Rest on the donor couch/chair for at least 10 minutes after the donation and get up from donor couch/chair only after you are told.

Advise for the nursing staff or technicians during or after blood collection:

1. Never leave a donor alone during blood donation. Always talk with donors to make them comfortable and anxiety free. Answer to their queries.
2. If you observe a vasovagal reaction—the feet to be raised, clothing's to be loosen and belt to be removed.
   a. Apply cool pack on the forehead of the donor.
   b. If vomiting is there, make the donor to a lateral position.
   c. If loss of consciousness is there for more than 60 sec, IV fluid may be required.
3. During donation, if donor faints, stop blood collection and remove the needle immediately. Make the head end of the couch/chair down or alternatively raise the donor legs and take aromatic ammonia spirit cotton just near the nose. Monitor blood pressure, pulse rate and temperature under the supervision of doctor (transfusion medicine or trained doctor).

Before starting the blood collection of a day, check routinely oxygen cylinder and emergency drugs as per directions of drugs and cosmetics rule.

Checklist for the nursing staff or technicians before blood collection:

- Check the donor number and identity from the donor questionnaire and blood bag
- Check the blood bag for leaks, breaks, turbidity or changes in colour of anticoagulant
- Anticoagulant should be clear.
- Check for any fungal growth over the bag or under the label.
- Check for needle seal and lock.

Blood collection/phlebotomy procedure:

- Donor should sit on the donor couch comfortably, spreading his/her arm on the arm-rest, exposing the arm (cubital fossa) without any tightness around the upper arm due to the folded shirt sleeve.
- Ensure that the donor is relaxed, ask him/her to watch TV/listen music during the blood donation.
- All relevant records like the donor's name, bag number, pilot tube number/bar code vacutainer, and name must be registered properly on the donor's card. The number on the blood bag and pilot test tubes/bar code vacutainer must tally with the donor's card.
- The blood bag should be thoroughly examined for leaks, cracks, or punctures. The anticoagulants must be inspected and it should be clear.
- The bag is to be kept over a bio-mixer or with spring balance or on a blood bag weighing machine.
- Apply a BP cuff/tunicate on the donor's arm.
- The median cubital vein inside the elbow which is close to the skin is chosen for blood donation. Locate the vein perfectly, feel it. A prominent one has to be chosen for phlebotomy (Fig. 4.1).

- Access that vein without any injury.
- Clean the vein using alcohol, and iodine then alcohol and dry the area.
- The quality of the needle should be very good (ISO 3826), remove the plastic cover on the phlebotomy needle and perform venipuncture immediately.
- The needle should be inserted gently into the vein to collect the blood.
- Advice the donor to continuously squeeze the hand roller to improve blood flow.
- Ensure proper mixing of blood and anticoagulant during blood collection. Adequate flow rate should be monitored.
- When the bag is filled with blood, the BP cuff is released, clamp the tube and the needle is removed gently from the donor's vein. Keep a cotton role on the venipuncture site, and apply pressure to prevent bleeding. After 10–15 minutes, look for the clot, and then a bandage is placed for the next few hours.
- The tube is clamped at two sites close to the donor side and sealed in the middle.
- Blood is collected in the pilot tubes or barcode vacutainer.
- Blood collection should be completed within 8–10 minutes.

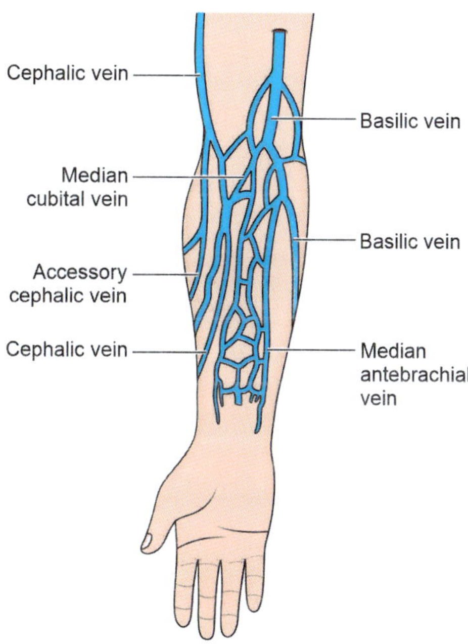

Fig. 4.1: Median cubital vein inside the elbow

Note:
Dr James Blundell, a British Obstetrician made the first blood transfusion of human blood in 1818 for the treatment of postpartum hemorrhage (PPH).
Always wear gloves while handling blood specimens.
An average healthy person has 5–6 L of blood in the body.

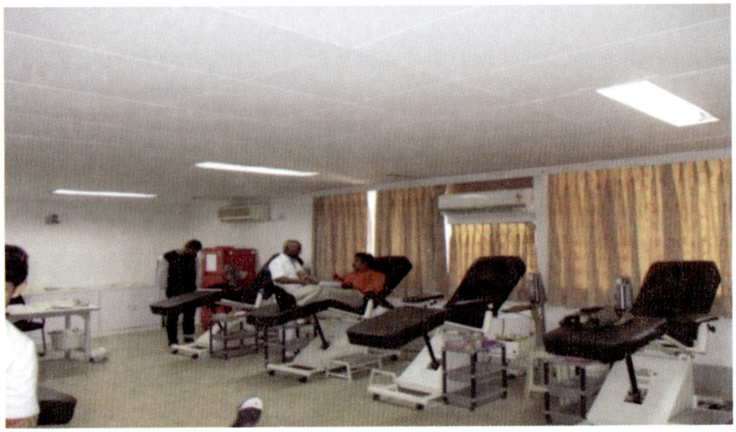

Fig. 4.2: Blood donation room blood donors are donating blood on donor couch

Post-Donation Care

- After blood donation the blood donor should be kept under close observation (Fig. 4.2).
- Immediately after blood donation, the adverse donor reactions may occur like syncope, vomiting, hyperventilation, and neuromuscular excitability like tetany, vasovagal reaction and bradycardia/hypotension. Rarely delayed syncope may occur after 30 minutes to 1 hour of donation. Medical officer should attend the donor.
- The donor should report to the blood centre physically or by phone if any feeling of dizziness, vomiting, blackening, giddiness after leaving the donor complex or hospital.
- To avoid any injury due to fall, donor should take rest for a duration of 30 minutes following blood donation.
- Donors should take adequate fluid to replenish the blood volume.
- Donors are advised to keep the cotton pressed over the phlebotomy site for 15–20 minutes till the bleeding stops. Then a band-aid is put on the phlebotomy site.
- Donors are advised not to do heavy work like jogging, dancing, gym and lifting heavy objects on the phlebotomy side hand.
- Donors are advised not to smoke for next 6 hr and consume alcohol on the day of blood donation.
- Donors are denied for driving after blood donation.
- If any hematoma occurs, compress the area with cotton to remove the extravasated blood and inform the donor about the occurrence of color change of the skin. The donor is advised to apply ice-pack on the site and if required thrombophob gel to manage the pain.
- The donor is advised to contact blood centre for any discomfort after leaving the premises.

Chapter 5

Components Preparation and Storage

MATERIALS REQUIRED FOR BLOOD COMPONENTS PREPARATION

- Double bags/triple bags and quadruple bags.
- Bucket (Fig. 5.1a)
- Scissors
- Pliers
- Forceps
- Plastic clips
- Rubber band
- Marker
- Plastic bar stick/rod stick and soft plastic pieces (Fig. 5.1b)
- Stripper (used to mix the blood component in the tubing with the bag)
- Gloves, cotton, and spirit.

Instrument Materials Required

- Blood bank refrigerator
- Refrigerated centrifuge
- Horizontal laminar air-flow bench
- Deepfreeze–40°C and –80°C
- Electronic or manual plasma expresser
- Weighing balance with double pan
- Electronic weighing machine (single pan)
- Di-electric tube sealer (Fig. 5.1c)
- Platelet agitator incubator
- Refrigerated circulating plasma
- Cryo-water bath
- Weighing scale
- Saline stand
- Blood group labels and component labels
- Biomedical waste disposal buckets with proper color codes.

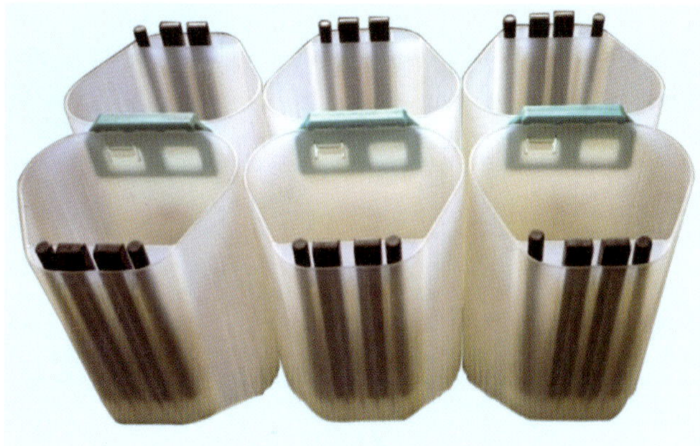

Fig. 5.1a: Buckets

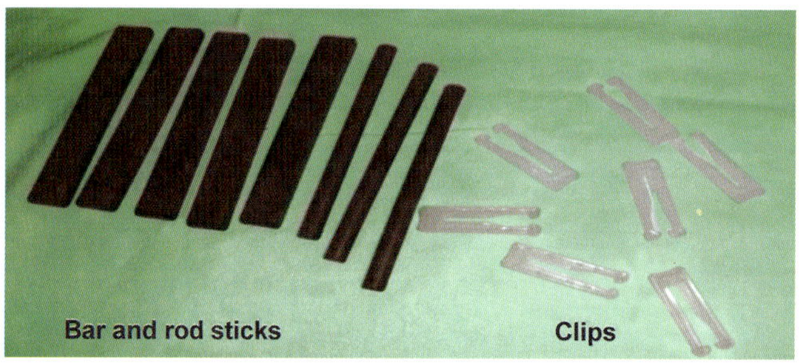

Fig. 5.1b: Bar, rod sticks, and clips

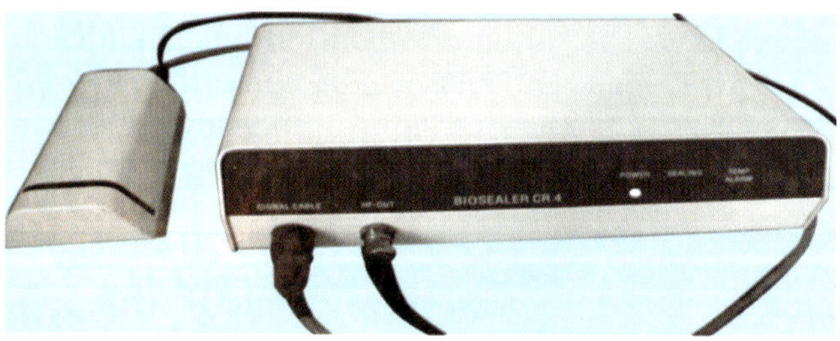

Fig. 5.1c: Di-electric tube sealer

Di-electric tube sealer is used for sealing blood bag segments and it helps to detach different component products.

BAG SELECTION

- For blood component preparation either by buffy coat method or platelet rich plasma (PRP) method, bag selection is very important.
- In general, 4 types of blood collection bags are used, viz. single bags, double bags, triple bags, and quadruple bags. Mother blood bag volume is either 350 ml or 450 ml. Usually 450 ml blood bag is preferred for adequate volume of platelet and plasma preparation.

- Special types of top-and-bottom bags are used for automated extractor machines and these bags are used for component preparation by buffy coat method.
- Special types of blood bags are made like:
  - Top and bottom blood bag with leukocyte filter.
  - Top and bottom quadruple/triple blood bag.
  - Top and top triple/quadruple blood bag.
  - Penta blood bag.

Top and bottom bag: The primary bag which collects the blood from a donor is also known as mother bag. This bag is connected to one satellite bag through its bottom which stores the packed red cell. Other satellite bags are attached to the mother bag from its top.

Top and top bag: All the satellite bags are connected to the mother bag through the top of the bags.

Top and bottom blood bag with leukocyte filter for red cells: Top and bottom penta blood bags with a filter for whole blood collection (450 ml, CPD/SAGM-2) and separation of three different blood components like leuko-depleted packed red cell, FFP, and platelets concentrate. (CPD: Citrate phosphate dextrose, SAGM: Saline, adenine, glucose, mannitol).

Top and bottom quadruple blood bag: Top and bottom quadruple blood bags for whole blood collection (450 ml, CPD/SAGM-2) and separation of three different blood components like leuko-depleted packed red cell, FFP, and platelets concentrate by buffy coat method.

Top and bottom triple blood bag: Top and bottom triple blood bags for whole blood collection (450 ml CPD/SAGM-2) and separation of two different blood components like leuko-depleted packed cell and FFP. And these bags are used for automated component preparation extractor machines.

Penta blood bag: Designed for pediatric/multiple transfusions. It reduces the risk of multiple donor exposure to pediatric patients. It prevents wastage of blood as one unit can be divided into five different parts.

Single blood bag with CPDA-1: Collect 350 ml of human blood for whole blood collection. The bag contains 49 ml CPDA-1 preservative solution and the life of the blood is 35 days (Fig. 5.2a).

Note: The ratio of CPDA-1 and blood is—IP 14 ml of CPDA-1 for 100 ml of whole blood.

Double blood bag with CPDA: Collect 350 ml of blood in a double bag, and the whole blood is separated into packed red cells (PRC) and plasma (FFP) through the process of centrifugation and extraction. In this bag 49 ml CPDA preservatives are available. The size of the plasma transfer satellite bag is the same as the primary bag (mother bag) (Fig. 5.2b). Life of the blood is 35 days.

Double blood bag with SAGM-2 bag: One mother bag contains IP49 ml CPD preservative solution for 350 ml of whole blood. One satellite bag is specially made for FFP preparation and 80 ml of SAGM-2 preservative is available in this bag. The size of the plasma transfer satellite bag is the same as the primary bag (mother bag). An extra two satellite pouches also connect in this bag for storage of SAGM2 and another for

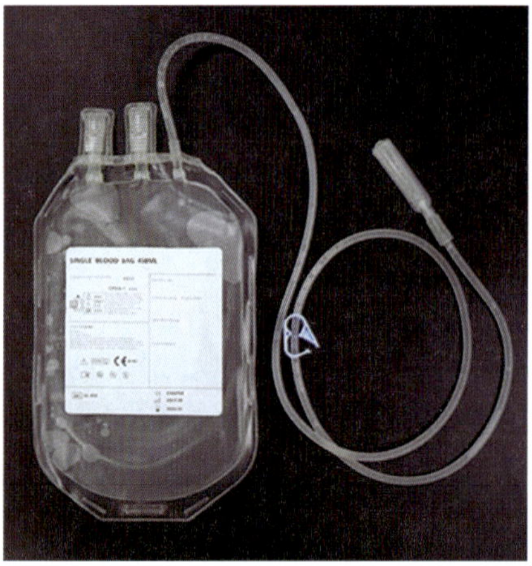

Fig. 5.2a: Single blood bag

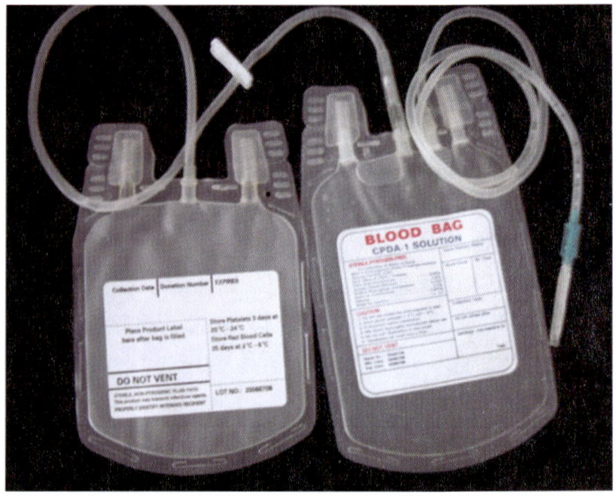

Fig. 5.2b: Double blood bags

buffy-coat (leucocytes) collection. The inclusion of an additive solution helps to extend the shelf life of the PRC to 42 days.

Triple blood bag with SAGM-2: The mother bag (primary bag) contains IP 63 ml CPD for the collection and preservation of 450 ml human blood and two satellite bags. The size of the two satellite bags is the same as the primary bag. One satellite bag contains 100 ml SAGM-2 additive solution for red blood cell preservation. One satellite bag is specially made for platelet concentrate preparation. The triple bags are used for three different types of component preparation PRC, FFP, platelets concentrate or cryoprecipitate component.

Quadruple blood bag with SAGM-2 preservative: The mother bag (primary bag) contains IP 63 ml CPD for the collection and preservation of 450 ml human blood and three satellite bag (Fig. 5.3). The size of the remaining two satellite bags is the same as the primary bag. One small transfer satellite bag made 100 ml of capacity for buffy-coat collection. One satellite bag contains 100 ml SAGM-2 additive solution for red blood cell preservation. One transfer satellite bag for storage of plasma (FFP) at

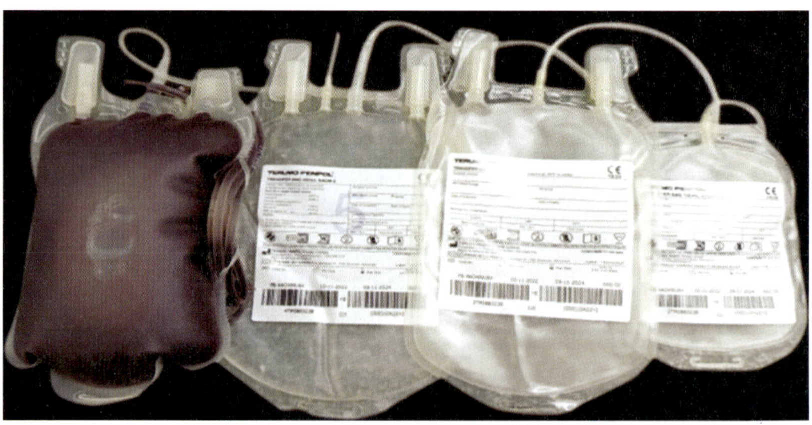

Fig. 5.3: Whole blood (450 ml) in quadruple bags

–40°C or colder. The quadruple bags are used for all types of component preparation like packed cell/leuko-depleted packed red cell, FFP, platelets concentrate through the buffy-coat method and cryoprecipitate component.

For the preparation of FFP, PRC, and random donor's platelets, 350 ml/450 ml of blood is collected in the anticoagulated bag of triple bags, and the satellite bags are used for the preparation of FFP and random donor platelets (Table 5.1).

An additional 80 ml SAGM-2 preservatives for 350 ml of the triple bag and double bag and 100 ml SAGM-2 preservatives for 450 ml of quadruple bag and triple bag are there. If SAGM-2 is used as a preservative, then the red cell life span is increased to 42 days. In quadruple/triple bags one satellite bag is specially made for platelet concentrate preparation.

Table 5.1: Different types of bag utilization for suitable blood components from blood donors of weight 45–55 kg and >55 kg

Donor details		*Components*	*Blood bag details*	
Weight of donor	*Taken aspirin*		*Type*	*Volume (ml)*
>55 kg	No	PRC + FFP + PC	Triple or quadruple	450 ml
>55 kg	Yes	PRC + FFP PRC + FFP/cryo	Double Triple	350 ml 450 ml
45–55 kg	No	PRC + FFP + PC PRC + FFP/cryo PRC + FFP	Triple Triple Double	350 ml
45–55 kg	Yes	PRC + FFP PRC + FFP/cryo	Double Triple	350 ml

FFP: Fresh frozen plasma, PRC: Packed red cell, PC: Platelet concentrate, Cryo: Cryoprecipitate

PRECAUTIONS REQUIRED FOR BLOOD COMPONENTS PREPARATION

The selection of areas, maintaining sterility, avoiding pollution hazards, and taking other precautions are very important for the quality of component preparation. Some instructions are given below.

Precautions for Blood Component Separation Unit

- The premises used for processing of blood components should be kept in a sterile, clean, and pollution-free area.
- As per the national guidelines, an additional 50 square meters in the blood centre is required for a blood component license.
- Room should be fully air-conditioned and temperature to be maintained at 20–24°C.
- Component preparation should always be in a closed system to maintain sterility and avoid contaminations.
- One changing room should be there for sterile precaution.
- Before entering in the preparation area change shoes and wear disposable gloves, gown, cap, musk, etc.
- Hot air oven, autoclave machine, incubator, tap water, basin, ceiling fan, wooden rack, etc. should not be placed in a component processing area.
- Out let drainage is not allowed.

Precautions during Blood Collection

- According to the components to be prepared from the blood unit, donor selection, health and weight of the donor, and selection of the bag are very important.
- Quality of the container and anticoagulant preservative solution should be maintained.
- The technique of phlebotomy should be appropriate.
- Before collection of blood clean the donor's vein with betadine solution and isopropyl alcohol to remove bacteria as much as possible.
- For blood component preparation during collection, blood should be mixed properly with respective anticoagulants by an automated shaker or gently shaken by hand.
- For blood component preparation, an accurate volume of blood should be collected (350/450 ± 10%) according to the anticoagulants supply in the bag. It should be strictly followed for a quality product.
- For optimum quality component preparation, 450 mL whole blood (WB) collection is preferred because optimum platelets yields and adequate plasma volume is available.
- During collection donor cuff pressure may be maintained at 40–70 mmHg for smooth blood flow.
- After the collection of blood, close the collection tubing by the pinch clamp and seal the collection tube with a di-electric sealer nearest to needle. Mix the blood in the tubing to the mother bag and then seal it into several segments with a di-electric sealer machine.
- According to the preparation of the respective component, check and ensure that the donor number and other records in the mother bag (primary bag) and satellite bags are the same. Donor details and component details should be documented on the component preparation register, master register.

Steps for Component Separation

- Preparation of the blood components should be completed within 6 hours of collection and particularly FFP should be stored at –80°C immediately after preparation.
- The blood unit is kept at room temperature (20°–24°C) for an hour in upright position to avoid red cell contamination of platelet.
- Keep the blood bag gently on the inner side of the bucket (surface of a plain narrow area) for an hour at room temperature (Fig. 5.5a). During this time RBC will be settled and production will be good. Keep the satellite bags in between the mother bag and collection tube with clips (locks) to prevent any damage to the blood bag during centrifugation.
- Stroke gently the tubing bottom and top of the bag by soft plastic stick bar (glass sealer and upper tube) to remove red cells which prevents red cell contamination platelet rich plasma after centrifugation.
- Before balancing the blood bag buckets, check the weighing machine (Fig. 5.4a) and place the bags at the center of the machine properly.
- Balance the blood bags with buckets (Fig. 5.5b); the weight of the opposite bucket should be equal.
- Accurate balance is done by plastic stick bar, plastic rod, and final adjustment by pieces of soft plastic.

- Place the blood bag bucket inside the refrigerated centrifuge diagonally (opposite). (Figs 5.6a to c).
- If only two bags of components are to be prepared, then two pair of buckets should be used. The blood bag buckets are always placed towards the center of the centrifuge and the empty buckets towards the centrifugation wall (both blood bags facing the same direction at the center of the centrifuge).
- Before running the refrigerated centrifuge, check all parameters according to the respective component program and leave it in running condition for half an hour.
- During this time, the compressor will start and help to reach the desired temperature.
- Components preparation is always done under a laminar airflow bench with sterile conditions to avoid bacterial contamination.
- Before and after the preparation of the component, clean the laminar air flow bench area.
- Plasma expresser, weighing balance (used for prepared component volume), di-electric tubing, sealer, plastic clips, marker, all materials are available inside the laminar bench during component preparation.
- Do not use plastic clips during centrifugation; the blood bag can be damaged or ruptured.
- Take out the respective component unit with buckets from the refrigerated centrifuge very carefully otherwise the segregation layer will be disturbed (plasma will be mixed with RBC).
- Take out the prepared unit bag from buckets very carefully; hold the upper seal of the mother bag (primary bag) by thumb and index finger very tightly. Then turn up without disturbance and place on plasma expresser.
- Before breaking the sealer of the mother bag, check all records like blood group, donor/unit number, name of the component, date of collection, and expiry, and also check leakage of the bag and for visible red cell on the top of the mother bag/ tubing. To settle down the red cells from the tubing, the blood bag is kept for a few minutes on the plasma expresser.
- During the preparation of the product if hemolysis is visible discard the plasma bag.
- During the preparation of the product if a hyperactive color is visible (pale yellow) and the plasma product is discarded. (Though routinely, bilirubin is not tested, if it is tested, the result shows more than 1.2 mg%.)
- After separating the respective components, seal the tube with a di-electric sealer at two or three respective distances.
- During the preparation of the respective component unit after completing the collection of plasma in the respective satellite bag, air must be released to the mother bag or extra empty satellite bag.
- After completing the preparation, paste the blood group label on the mother bag and the respective components label on the component bags and keep it according to the storage temperature.
- Document the details of the blood component, i.e. donor unit number, segment number, date of collection (DOC), date of expiry of each component (DOE), the volume of the component, blood group, TTI screening status, etc. in the component preparation register and master register.

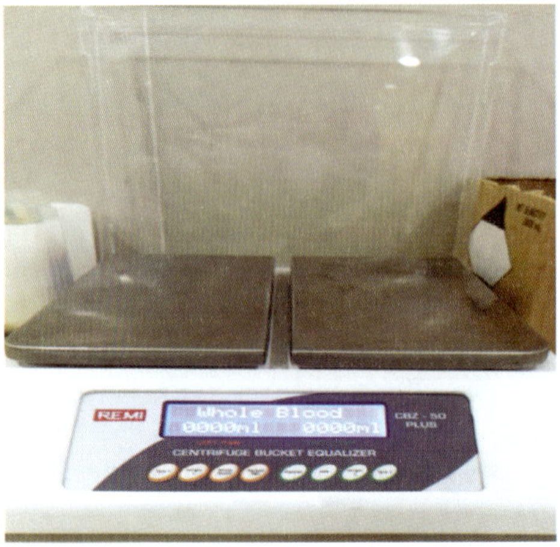

Fig. 5.4a: Double pan weighing balance

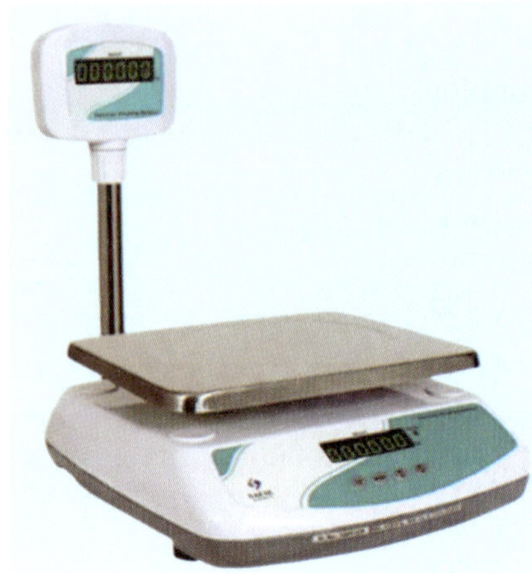

Fig. 5.4b: Single pan weighing scale

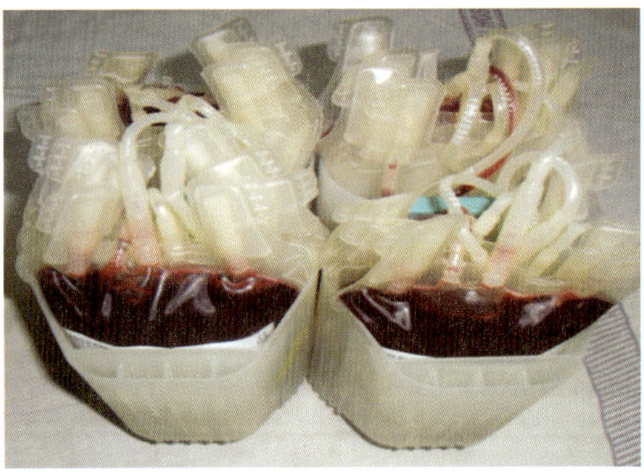

Fig. 5.5a: Blood bags in buckets

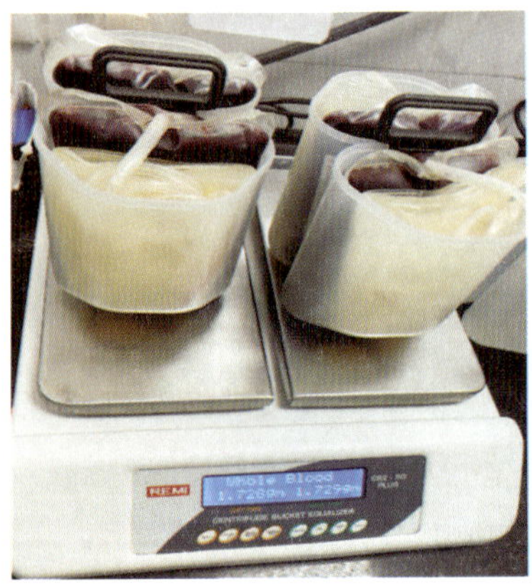

Fig. 5.5B: Weighing balance with blood bags buckets

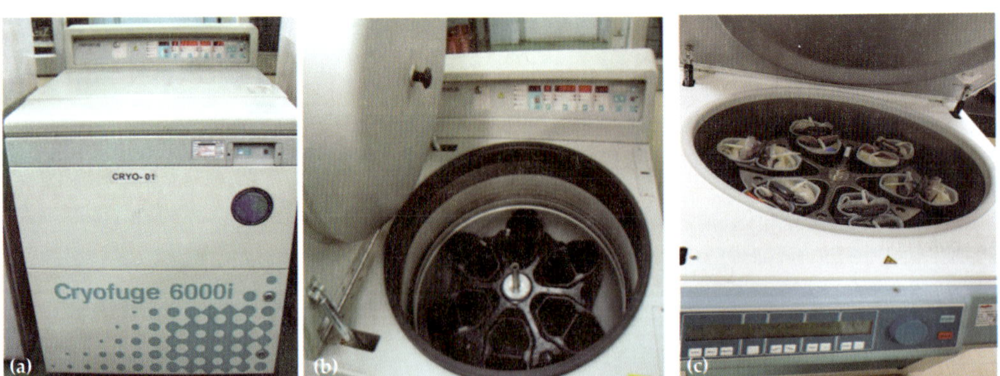

Figs 5.6a to c: (a and b) Refrigerated blood bag centrifuge, (c) Balanced blood bags in the bucket

DIFFERENT METHODS OF BLOOD COMPONENT PREPARATION

For blood components preparation mainly two spins are used, i.e. 'light spin and hard spin'. To separate packed red blood cells (PRC)/leuko-depleted packed blood cells from fresh frozen plasma (FFP) in double bag, and cryoprecipitate from FFP only 'hard spin' is used. Depending on the sequence of spin, there are basically two different methods of random donor platelet RDP blood component preparation.

1. Platelet rich plasma (PRP) method
2. Buffy coat method

Platelet Rich Plasma (PRP) Method

WB collected in triple/quadruple bag is centrifuged with soft spin (1500–2000 g force) first to separate the PRP and PRC; followed by hard spin (5000 g force) to the PRP bag to prepare RDP and FFP, as shown in Flowchart 5.1a.

Flowchart 5.1a: Blood component preparation by PRP method

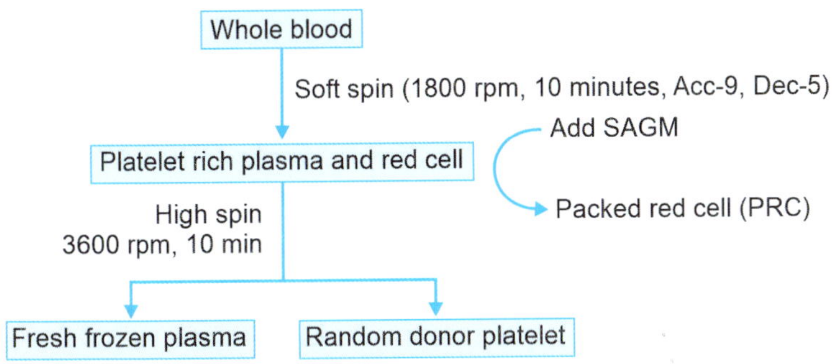

Buffy Coat Method

Unlike that of the PRP method, in the buffy coat (BC) method, the WB is centrifuged with hard spin (5000 g force) first to separate PRC and FFP from the buffy coat followed by soft spin (1500–2000 g force) to the buffy coat to prepare the RDP.

Flowchart 5.1b: Blood component preparation by BC method

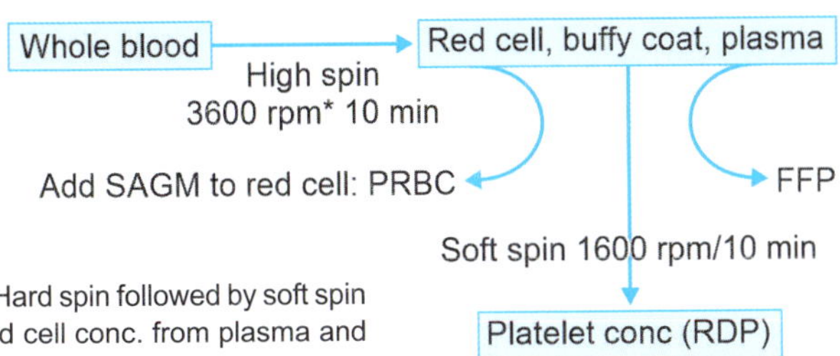

* **Buffy coat method:** Hard spin followed by soft spin is given to separate red cell conc. from plasma and buffy coat (platelet)

Blood Component Separation Programs of the Refrigerated Centrifuge

There are different manufacturers for the blood bag refrigerated centrifuge (BBRC) and their capacity, rotor size radius is different. Each manufacturer sets the program for different blood component preparation, in such a manner that the product yield will be maximum. Depending on the blood bag type/volume, the program is different in the form of centrifugation/rotation per minute (RPM), acceleration, deceleration, and duration of centrifugation. Temperature also differs in each program depending on the blood component prepared. Some examples of program for PRP or BC method blood component preparation is summarized in Table 5.2. The program differs w.r.t institute also with the same manufacturer.

Table 5.2: Examples of different program in refrigerated centrifuge with the temperature, acceleration, deceleration, RPM, and duration

Program number	*Method*	*Temp in C*	*Acelrn*	*Decelrn*	*RPM*	*Duration (min)*
PRP-SS1	350 ml (PRP-soft spin)	22	9	3	1400	10
PRP-SS2	450 ml (PRP-soft spin)	22	9	3	1400	12
PRP-HS3	350/450 ml PRP hard spin	22	6	4	3600	10
BC1	Buffy coat hard spin	22	9	3	3400	6
BC2	Buffy coat soft spin	22	8	4	600	6
CP1	Cryoprecipitate	4	6	4	3600	10

Platelet (RDP) Preparation

The platelet concentrate (RDP) is prepared either by PRP or BC method, accordingly the program of the centrifuge differs. Before centrifuging PRP bag or BC bag, the BBRC should be pre-run with the desired program to achieve the required temperature (22°C). During the preparation of RDP, keep the buffy-coat bag or PRP bag inside the buckets in a vertical position and packing should be appropriate in buckets with empty blood bags (transfer bag)/thermocol to prevent stacking of the bag. Because the volume of buckets is much larger compared to the volume of above product in bags. In PRP method, the PRP bag is centrifuged immediately after the separation from PRC, while in buffy coat method after the hard spin, PRC and plasma is separated from BC and the BC is kept hanging for 4–6 hours before centrifugation for RDP preparation.

Cryoprecipitate Preparation

For the preparation of PRC/FFP/cryoprecipitate, the desired temperature is 4°C. Hence, before centrifuging the thawed FFP (at 4°C in cryobath, Fig. 5.7 or blood bank refrigerator, BBR), the BBRC is pre-run with the desired program to attend the required temperature. The plasma bag is kept in one bucket and extra satellite bag inside the other attached bucket. The same should be followed for the opposite balancing bucket. The above four bags will not be kept together inside a single bucket. Sometime two plasma bags are kept in a single bucket for appropriate packing or the packing should be with thermocol/transfer bag to prevent folding of plasma bags (or else plasma bags will be settled at the bottom and there may be mixing of plasma and cryoprecipitate which not let the separation of cryoprecipitate). After separation of cryo-poor plasma by plasma expresser, remaining 15–20 ml plasma with white precipitate (cryoprecipitate) is stored at –80°C and the life span is 1 year.

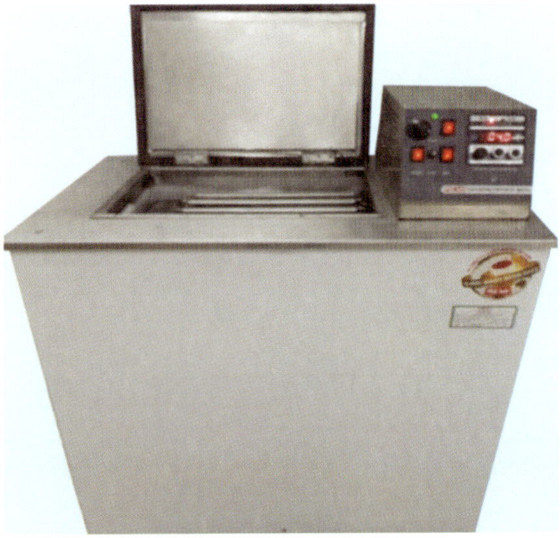

Fig. 5.7: Cryobath with 4°C temperature

Blood Component Preparation using Double Bags, Triple Bags and Quadruple Blood Bags

Double Bags

Double bags are either of two bags (mother and satellite bags) [type 1] or along with these SAGM and BC bag [type 2, Fig. 5.8]. The double bags are used to prepare PRC and FFP, as shown in Flowcharts 5.2a and 5.2b. Hard spin is given to separate the PRC from FFP (Figs 5.9a and b). While in the type 2 bag, upper plasma is separated into plasma bag and then buffy coat is separated manually into small buffy coat bag (discussed in detailed in quadruple bag). Then the SAGM is added to the PRC and the bag is sealed and separated.

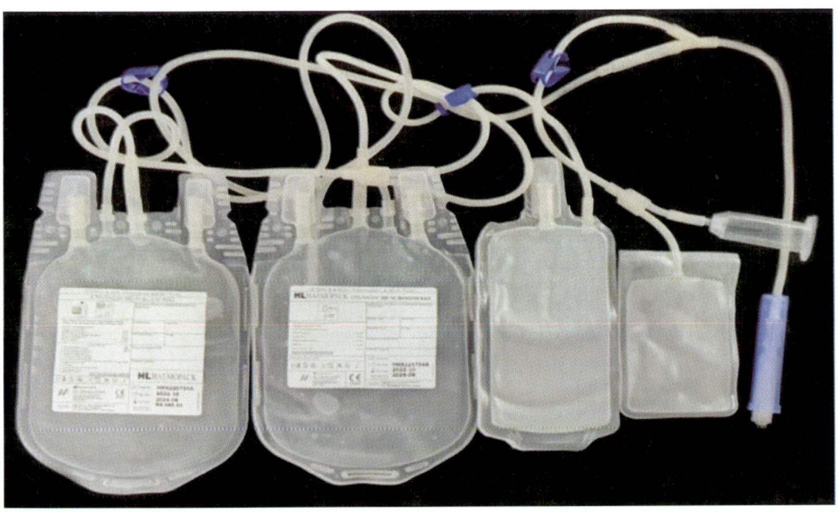

Fig. 5.8: Double bags with SAGM and small buffy coat bag

Flowchart 5.2a: PRC and FFP preparation using double bags

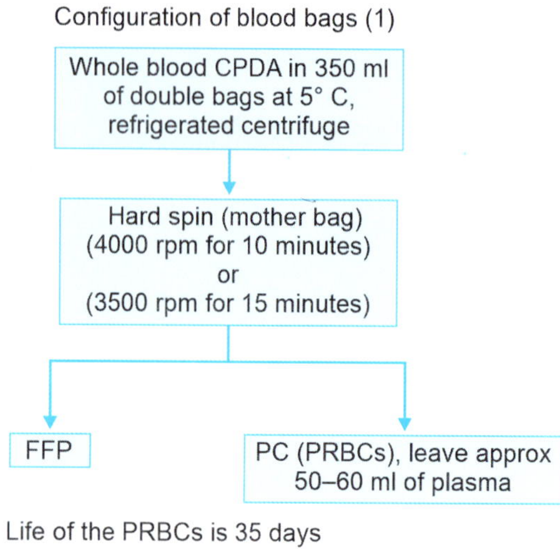

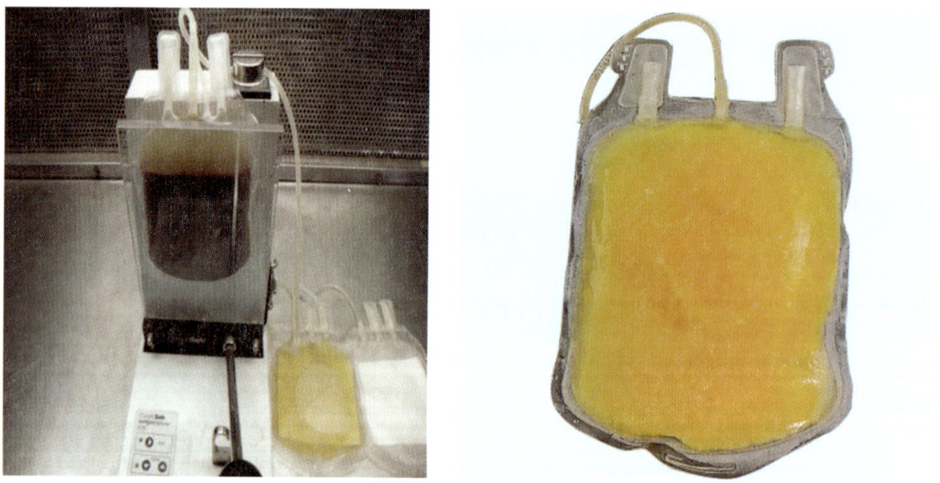

Fig. 5.9a and b: Plasma expressor separating PRC and FFP

Triple Bag

Triple bag (350/450 ml) is utilized to prepare PRC, FFP and RDP by PRP method or to prepare PRC and FFP/cryoprecipitate using hard spin program (Flowchart 5.3b and Fig. 5.10). The program of the refrigerated centrifuge is followed as per the desired component preparation is given in Table 5.2.

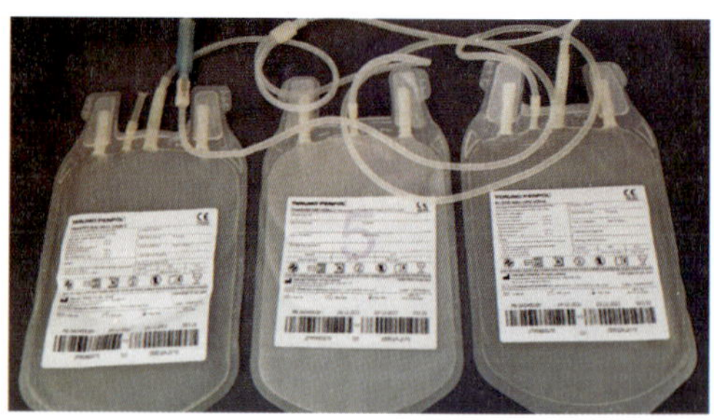

Fig. 5.10: Triple bag (mother bag, SAGM bag and empty platelet bag)

In the PRP method (Flowchart 5.3a) WB is centrifuged with soft spin, red cell will be settled down at the bottom and PRP remains on top. The bag is removed from

Flowchart 5.2b: Leukodepleted-PRC and FFP preparation using double bag

Configuration of blood bags (2)

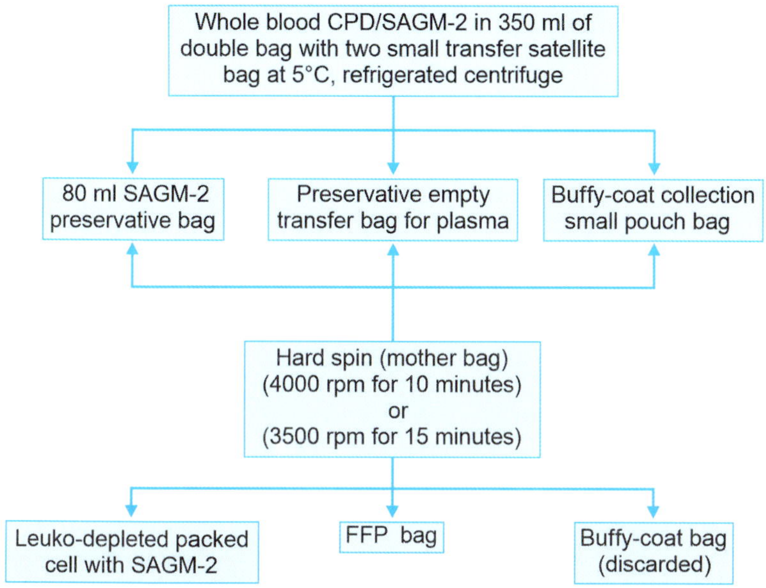

Life of the PRBCs is 42 days

the centrifuge without disturbing the separating layers and kept in the plasma expressor. The glass seal at the top of the mother bag is broken to separate the PRP into the RDP bag. Then the seal of the SAGM bag is broken to add the SAGM to red cell (PRC). PRP bag is centrifuged with hard spin (desired program). Platelet will be settled down and the platelet poor plasma is separated into the empty bag (SAGM) leaving 50–70 ml plasma to suspend the platelet. Plasma is stored at –80°C and termed as FFP. This platelet concentrate is termed as RDP.

Flowchart 5.3a: PRC, FFP and RDP preparation using triple bag

Configuration of blood bags (1)

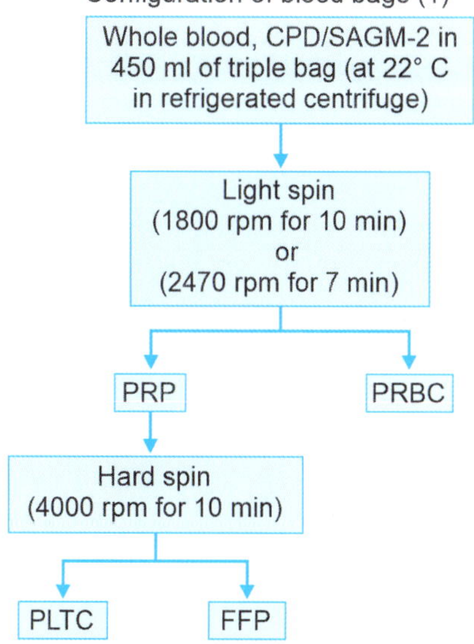

Cryoprecipitate Preparation using Triple Bag

WB is centrifuged with hard spin (desired program), to separate PRC from FFP as described above. Clamp the connecting tube between plasma bag and empty satellite bag. FFP along with the empty bag (SAGM) is stored in the deep freezer at –80°C or –40°C. Take out the solid plasma bag marked as cryoprecipitate from deep freeze and keep at room temperature for 5–10 minutes (during this time bag will be soft; if it is hard there will be possibility of breakage) and thaw at 4°C circulating cryo-water bath or at 4°C cold room/blood bank refrigerator. It will take 30–45 minutes to thaw. These FFP (cryo) bags are packed in the bucket appropriately using transfer bag/thermocol to prevent stacking of the bags. Then the bags are balanced and centrifuged using desired program to separate cryo-poor plasma from cryoprecipitate (Flowchart 5.3b).

Flowchart 5.3b: PRC, FFP and cryoprecipitate from FFP preparation using triple bags

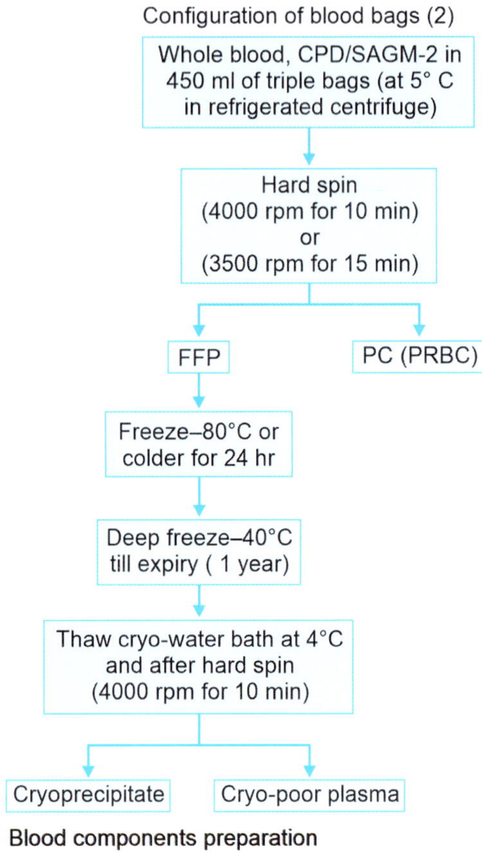

Quadruple Bag (*Fig. 5.11*)

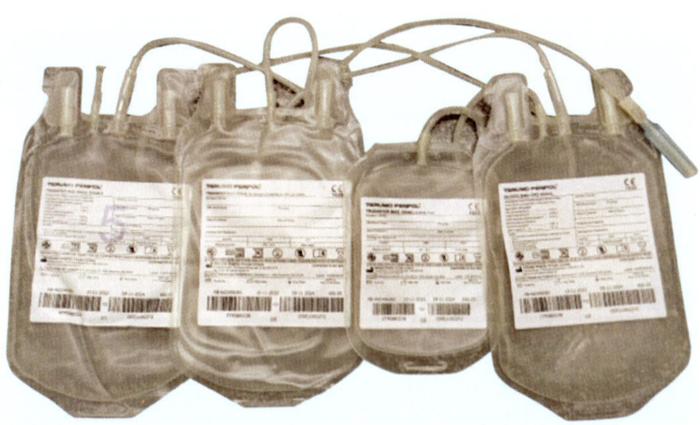

Fig. 5.11: Quadruple bag (mother bag, SAGM bag and empty platelet bag and plasma bag)

Preparation of PRC, RDP, FFP/Cryoprecipitate Using Quadruple Bag

Using PRP method, PRC is separated from PRP by soft spin (desired program). (Flowchart 5.4a) PRP is centrifuged with hard spin (desired program) to separate RDP from plasma. Plasma stored at –80°C and then thawed at 4°C to prepare cryoprecipitate, as discussed above.

Flowchart 5.4a: PRC, RDP, FFP/cryoprecipitate preparation using quadruple bag

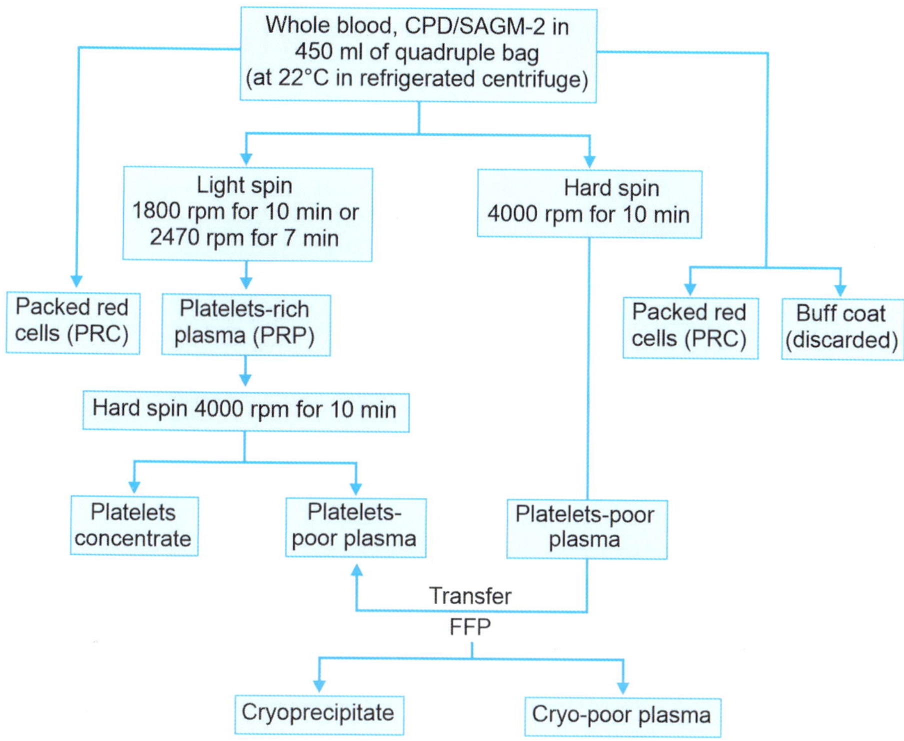

Preparation of Leukoreduced-PRC, RDP, FFP Using Quadruple Bag

WB is centrifuged with hard spin (desired program), to create three layers, red cell at bottom, plasma at top and the buffy coat in the middle. The bag is removed from the bucket without disturbing the layers and kept on the plasma expressor (Fig. 5.12a). The glass seal of the mother bag and empty plasma bag is broken to separate the plasma into the plasma bag and clamp the connecting tube.

Then the buffy coat layer is manually separated from red cells into the empty bag (Figs 5.12b to e). Squeeze or press surface of the buffy-coat area by finger very carefully and transfer maximum amount of buffy-coat with 15 to 20 ml of RBCs. After collection clamp immediately mother bag tubing connector by plastic clip (near Y connector). Remove clamp from the FFP bag end tubing and squeeze it to release air with transferring a little amount of plasma in to buffy-coat plasma bag (4th satellite bag). This plasma will help to clean the connected tubing area containing the RBCs and buffy-coat. Then clamp the tubing of the buffy-coat plasma bag by a plastic clip. Seal the plasma (FFP) bag tubing by sealer and detach FFP bag from the mother bag. Add SAGM-2 preservative

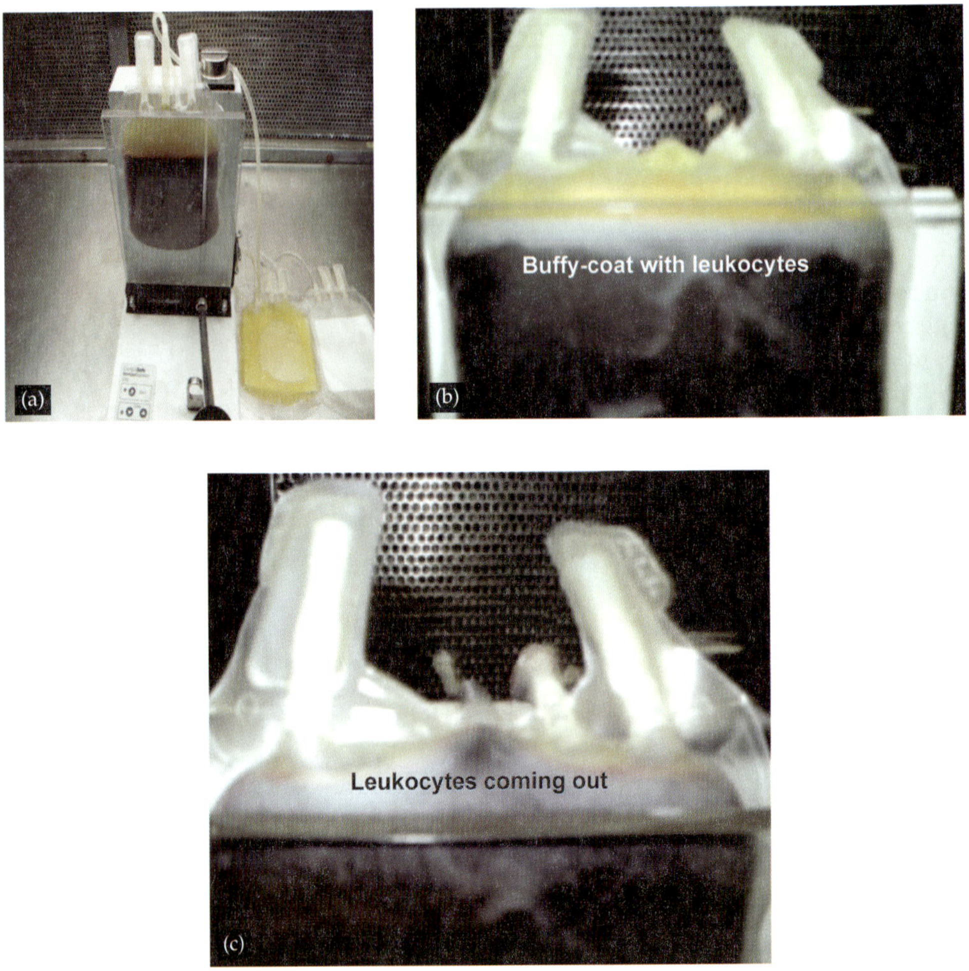

Figs 5.12a to c: (a) Plasma is separated from the buffy coat (middle layer) and red cell conc. (b) Buffy coat layer (white color layer) above the red cell conc. (c) Buffy coat layer is being separated from red cell conc.

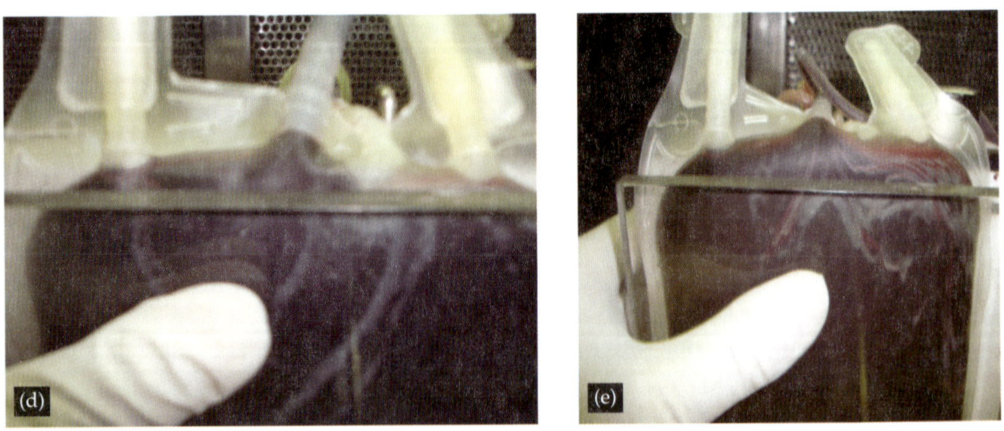

Figs 5.12d and e: Manual sqeezing of the blood bag to separate the buffycoat from red cell conc.

to mother bag and seal the connecting tube and separate the two. The final volume of plasma is approximately 200 ml, then store it at –80°C or lower for 24 hours. After that it is stored in deep freezer at –40°C till expiry.

Now the empty SAGM bag labeled as RDP, and buffy-coat collection satellite bag is hanged for 4–6 hr with the empty bag in an upward direction and the buffy-coat plasma bag in a downward position. During this time RBCs and buffy-coat will settle at the bottom. Buffy-coat bag and connected empty preservative bag are placed again inside the bucket and kept in a balanced manner. The buffy-coat bags are packed inside the buckets in a vertical position (without fold) using thermocol/transfer bag. Because during centrifugation buffy-coat plasma bag will be folded and settled at the bottom and there may be a chance of mixing or contamination. Buffy coat is centrifuged at light/soft spin (desired program) and then removed from the bucket without any disturbance to the layers. The BC bags are kept on the plasma expressor, clamp/rubber band over the connecting tube is removed and the platelet with plasma is transferred to the RDP bag. Buffy-coat bag will be discarded. The available volume of RDP is 70–90 ml in this method of RDP preparation.

(If platelet concentrate is not desired to prepare, the empty bag with FFP is stored to prepare cryoprecipitate as discussed above) (Flowchart 5.4b).

Flowchart 5.4b: PRC, FFP, and cryoprecipitate preparation using quadruple bag

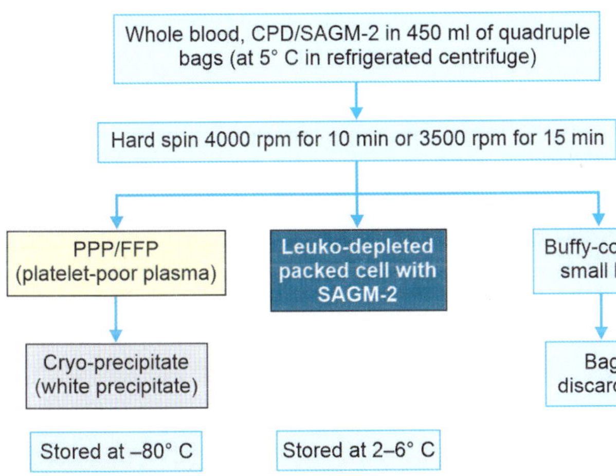

Storage of Blood Components

- Whole blood or PRC is stored in the blood bank refrigerator (Fig. 5.13) at 4°C. These units should be stored in vertical position and in a sequential manner so as to follow the first in first out policy easily.
- Due to heavy centrifugation, platelets are aggregated at the bottom of the bag. Hence it is necessary to keep the RDP units on the working surface till the aggregates dissolve. Platelets are resuspended by gently mixing and kept at 22–24°C in a platelet incubator with agitator (Fig. 5.14) until issue. Never keep the RDP units in an over lapping manner. Platelets are kept separately from each other and the plane surface being upward to allow them for proper oxygenation.

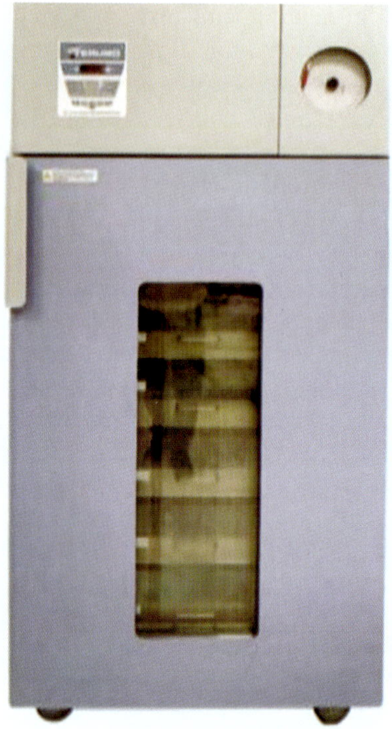

Fig. 5.13: Blood bank refrigerator

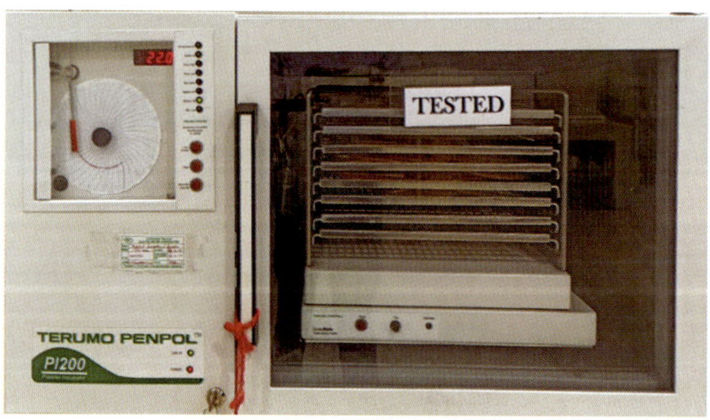

Fig. 5.14: Platelet agitator-incubator

- Platelet agitator-incubator should be calibrated in regular interval to maintain the temperature at 20–22°C and the agitation at 60–72/minutes. Reddish tinge of the concentrate indicates red cell contamination. There should be no grossly visible platelets aggregates during the storage. The swirling phenomenon should be checked before the issue. Shelf-life of platelets is 5 days from time of whole blood collection.
- Fresh frozen plasma is stored in deep freezer at –80°C (Fig. 5.15) and then transferred into –40°C. Cryoprecipitate also stored in same manner. Both have a life span of one year.

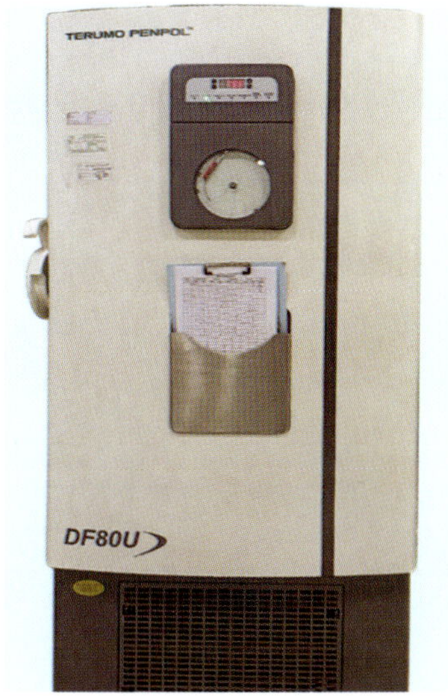

Fig. 5.15: Deep freezer

- Table 5.3 depicts the storage conditions of the blood components and their life span.

Table 5.3: Storage temperature, required equipment for different blood components and the life span

Blood component	*Storage equipment*	*Storage temperature*	*Life span*
Whole blood	Blood bank refrigerator	2–4°C	35 days
PRBC	Blood bank refrigerator	2–4°C	42 days
FFP	Deep freezer	–40°C/–80°C	1 year
RDP/SDP	Platelet agitator cum incubator	20–24°C	5 days
Cryoprecipitate	Deep freezer	–40°C/–80°C	1 year
Saline washed PRBC*	Blood bank refrigerator	Should be used within 6 hrs	
Leuko reduced PRBC**	Blood bank refrigerator	Same as PRBC	
Irradiated PRBC***	Blood bank refrigerator	Within 14 days	

Modification of blood components is required to prevent allergic reaction*, febrile nonhemolytic transfusion reaction**, and transfusion associated graft vs host disease***

Note:
- One healthy donor can donate up to 8 ml/kg body weight of blood safely.
- Adequate platelet yield and leukoreduced platelet is obtained by buffy coat method platelet preparation using a quadruple bag. Hence platelet preparation in this method is more preferred over triple bag/PRP method.
- Platelet yield from a 450 ml blood bag should be $>4.5 \times 10^{10}$/unit
- FFP preparation using blast freezer, freezes plasma more rapidly and hence provides increased yields of cryoprecipitate.
- An approved microwave thawing device maintaining 37°C should only be used for thawing plasma, not in any warm water or tap water.

Chapter 6

Advance Techniques of Blood Components Preparation

The word "Automation" is derived from the Greek word "Automatos" which means "acting of itself". Automation is introduced for the blood component separation unit to:

1. Increase the efficiency
2. Reduce the error
3. Reduce the risk of red cell contamination in platelets and FFP.
4. Maintain a similar volume of FFP and RDP

There are two types of automatic component separation machines:

1. **Automatic component extractor:** Whole blood is centrifuged like that of manual component separation, then the role of automatic component extractor comes.
2. **Automated whole blood processing:** Here, the whole blood is processed to PRBC and FFP, but the buffy-coat has to be pooled manually to extract the pooled platelet.

AUTOMATIC COMPONENT EXTRACTOR SYSTEM (ACS)

Special types of blood bags such as:

- Top and bottom (TAB) penta blood bag with leukocyte filter for PRBC
- Top and bottom (TAB) quadruple blood bag
- Top and bottom triple blood bag
- Top and top quadruple blood bag including one small 100 ml of buffy-coat collection satellite bag.

These blood bags are specially designed bags to be directionally used for the automatic component extractor (Fig. 6.1a and b). This machine is very scientific and accurate in order to achieve the most reliable and quality product. This automatic component extractor machine is commercially available and manufactured by different manufacturers.

PREPARATION OF DIFFERENT COMPONENTS FROM WHOLE BLOOD COLLECTED IN TOP AND BOTTOM PENTA BLOOD BAGS WITH LEUKOCYTE RC (RED CELL) FILTER

Principle

The same procedure for collecting whole blood is followed and then the unit is centrifuged with hard spin to create three layers such as red cells, buffy coat, and plasma. Then the ACS machine separates the unit into three different blood components, such as plasma, leuko-depleted packed cells and platelets concentrate.

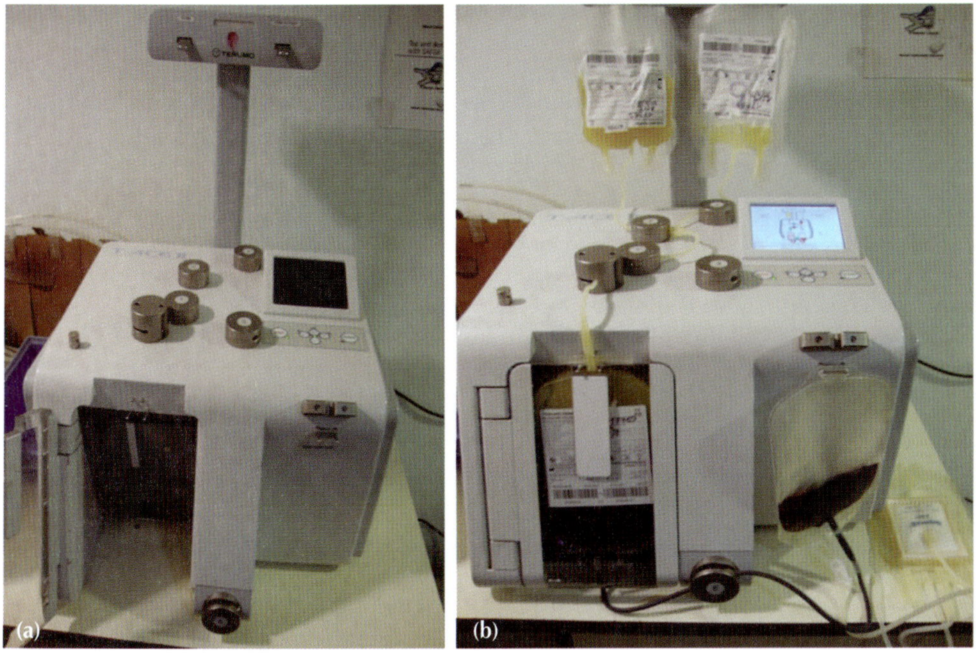

Fig. 6.1a and b: Automated component separation machine

Penta Bags Contain

- Mother bag: Contains CPD solution
- Plasma bag
- Satellite bag: Connected with a RC filter
- Platelet bag.

The mother bag is attached to the plasma and platelet bag at the top, while the transfer bag with leuko filter and SAGM-2 bag is attached to the bottom of the mother bag (Fig. 6.2).

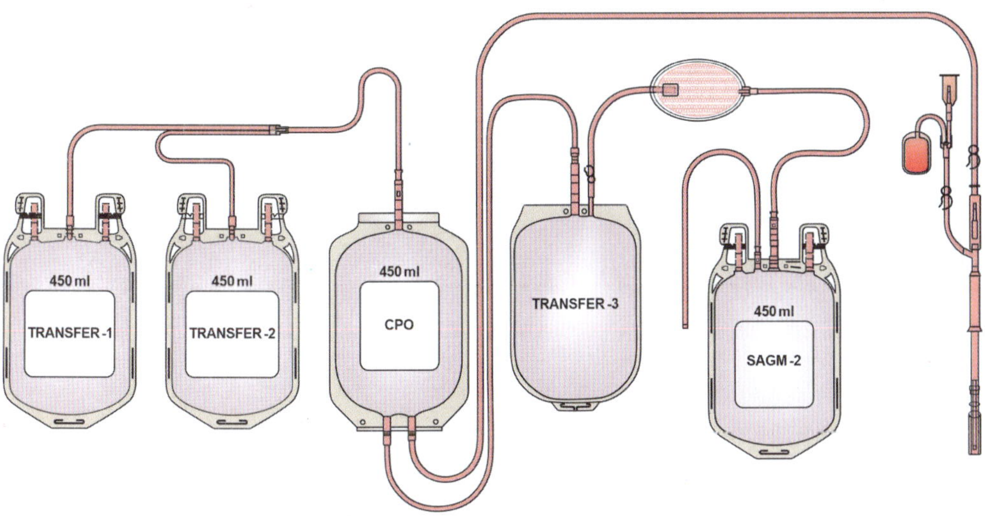

Fig. 6.2: Top and bottom bag with leukocyte filter for RBC

Step 1

Centrifugation Technique

- Collect appropriate volume of blood 450 ml in CPD penta blood bags system (donor bag contains 63 ml of anticoagulant, one satellite bag contains 100 ml of SAGM-2 preservative).
- The remaining satellite bag is already marked for platelets, platelets poor plasma (FFP) and leuko-depleted red blood cells collection.
- After collection of blood, store at room temperature (20–24°C) for one hour for settling the red cells to reduce the risk of red cell contamination of RDP.
- Keep the mother bag inside the bucket gently. Keep remaining satellite bags, leuko filter, connecting tubes and extra preservative bag inside the attached bucket in a rolled manner. In a similar method, keep a balanced blood bag in the opposite bucket.
- Before taking weight of blood bag buckets check weight balance (electronic or monopan).
- Balance the blood bags with a bucket on the monopan weight balance or electronic weighing machine.
- Weight of the opposite buckets should be equal.
- In order to balance the blood bags in a bucket, use the small plastic bar and plastic rod and adjust minutely with soft plastic pieces.
- Before placing blood bag buckets inside the refrigerated centrifuge, check the temperature of the refrigerated centrifuge, and start the pre-run for program. During this time the required temperature reaches 22°C. RPM, ACCL, DECL, and TIME can be changed according to need because these parameters may differ from centrifuge to centrifuge.
- Place the blood bag buckets of the refrigerated centrifuge diagonally in opposite positions.
- Close the lid of the refrigerated centrifuge, if present, and select the appropriate program on the centrifuge as per the need of the component prepared. Refer to Chapter 5 for the application of the centrifugation speed, time, and temperature required to be given for the desired component.
- Start the refrigerated centrifuge at 'hard spin', (5000 g force, desired program).
- [RPM, acceleration, deceleration, and duration of centrifugation may change according to the program from centrifuge to centrifuge].
- After centrifugation open the lid and take out the bags from the bucket.
- Hard spin results in three layers inside the mother bag. The top layer is plasma without platelet, i.e. called platelets poor plasma (PPP). The middle layer contains a buffy- coat and the bottom layer contains red blood cell concentration.
- Important instruction—no sharp object should be placed during centrifugation along with the blood bags. If the plastic clump is in use then use it with care, i.e. it should not be in contact with the blood bags.

Separation Technique

- Open the chamber window of the automatic component extractor machine and place the mother bag inside the chamber on a hanger. Do not disturb the layers, while placing the mother bag on a hanger without any turbulence. Then close the window.

- Hang red blood cells and the empty satellite bag on the hanger which is on the right side in the horizontal direction at 180° angle according to the manual instruction (this bag has no label).
- Hang the empty satellite bag (PPP collection) on the hanger over the mother bag according to the manual instruction.
- Hang the platelet satellite bag on a hanger over the red blood cells transfer bag according to the manual instruction.
- Keep the SAGM-2 preservative bag with the attached CRC filter on the machine desk table or hang it on the hanger according to the instruction.
- Place satellite bag tubing inside the channel clump cum sealer according to the manual instruction.
- Respective satellite bags should hang on the hanger according to the manufacturer's manual instruction, because these positions may differ from machine to machine.
- Before starting the machine, check thoroughly the automated component separation extractor as per manual instruction.
- Select the program as per manual instruction.
- Immediately break the mother bag and red cells transfer the satellite bag manually and start the machine.
- Now initially 5–10 ml top layer plasma comes from the mother bag automatically upwards direction through connecting tube and is stored ina platelet collection satellite bag. This plasma will help to remove red cells present in click tips. By doing this we get plasma without contamination and it is used for buffy-coat dilution or tubing clean during platelets concentration preparation.

  The machine will stop automatically as per programming.
- Remaining top layer plasma comes automatically from the mother bag is transferred in an empty satellite (PPP) collection bag through the connecting tube while the red cell layer is transferred into the bottom bag present in the downward position through the connecting tube.
- After completion of the plasma collection and red cells collection, the buffy-coat remains in the mother bag. A few ml of plasma will drip down from the PPP collection satellite bag and mix automatically with the buffy coat.
- Manually clamp the tubing of the platelet collection satellite bag.
- Plasma bag (PPP) and red cells transfer bag will be sealed automatically.
- ACS system will stop automatically as per programming.
- The volumel of plasma level varies and it depends on the donor's packed cell volume.
- Detach the plasma (PPP) bag from the remaining satellite bags.
- Detach red cells transfer bag from mother bag and platelets collection bag.
- Now the buffy-coat bag is already attached to the platelet collection bag.

  The red cells transfer bag is attached with SAGM-2 and RC filter bag (leuko-filter).
- Store platelet poor plasma (PPP) bag at –80°C or –40°C deep freeze for one year and this plasma should use as fresh frozen plasma or cryoprecipitate component.

Platelets Concentration Preparation by Buffy-coat Method (Fig. 6.3)

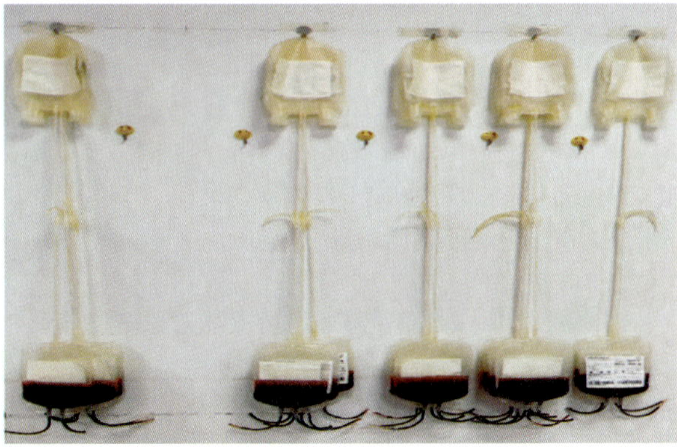

Fig. 6.3: PLTC preparation by buffy-coat method

Step II

- Hang the platelet collection bag along with the buffy-coat bag on the hangar for 4–6 hours. Hang the platelet collection bag at the top of the hanger keeping the buffy-coat plasma bag in a downward position as shown in Fig. 6.3. Remove the clamp from the platelet bag and release the 5–10 ml plasma which was transferred from the mother bag initially. This plasma will help to clean red cells in between connected tubing areas. During this time red cells and buffy-coat will settle at the bottom.
- Again clamp the tubing with soft plastic, to prevent the flow of plasma from the buffy-coat bag during centrifugation.
- Buffy-coat bag and connected platelets collection satellite bag are placed again inside the bucket gently and balance these bags by electronic weight machine.

Centrifugation Technique

Keep the buffy-coat bag inside the buckets in a vertical position (without fold).

During centrifugation, the buffy-coat plasma bag will be folded and settled at the bottom and there may be a chance of mixing or contamination. To prevent this, packing should be done in buckets with thermocol because the volume of buckets is too larger for the volume of buffy-coat with plasma.

- Start the refrigerated centrifuge at 'light spin' (1500–2000 g force, desired program).
- After centrifugation take out the bag from the bucket very carefully.
- 'Light spin' results in two layers; the top layer is platelets concentrate and the bottom layer is the remaining buffy-coat.

Separation Technique

Open the chamber window of the automatic component extractor system and keep the buffy-coat bag on the hanger. Hang empty platelets collection satellite bag on a hanger on the right side (horizontal direction at 1800 angle) according to the manual instruction. Place satellite bag tubing inside the channel clump cum sealer according to the manual instruction.

Before starting the system remove the soft plastic clamp manually from the transferring tube.

The top layer of platelet concentrate will be transferred to the platelet collection satellite bag. Seal platelets bag connected tubing automatically by sealer and detach from buffy-coat.

Manual Separation Technique

Keep the buffy-coat plasma bag on the plasma expresser and remove the rubber clamp from the connecting tube.

Transfer the platelet conc into the platelet bag and seal the platelet concentrate connected tubing by sealer and detach from the buffy-coat.

- Buffy-coat bag will be discarded. After the preparation of platelet concentrates (available volume is 50–60 ml), keep RDP inside the agitator incubator. Continuous agitation of 70–72 strokes/minute should be maintained throughout the storage period.

Leukocyte Poor Packed Cell Preparation by CRC Filter

Step III

Hang the SAGM-2 bag on a hanger at the top (mark as SAGM-2 packed cell) and keep the red cell bag at the bottom. Break the seal from the SAGM-2 bag and release the preservative through CRC filter to the red cell bag (Fig. 6.4).

- After complete drainage of the preservative, hang SAGM-2 with red cells bag at the top and empty the SAGM-2 bag in a downward direction.
- Wait for a few minutes for the complete transfer of red cell through CRC filter.
- Seal the tubing with a sealer and detach the leuko reduced PRBC from CRC filter.
- Satellite bag and CRC filter will be discarded.
- Blood bags should be stored in a vertical position at 2–6°C in the blood bank refrigerators for 42 days.
- Steps and procedure of blood component preparation may differ from machine to machine (automated) and it should follow manufacturer's manual instruction and blood centre SOP.

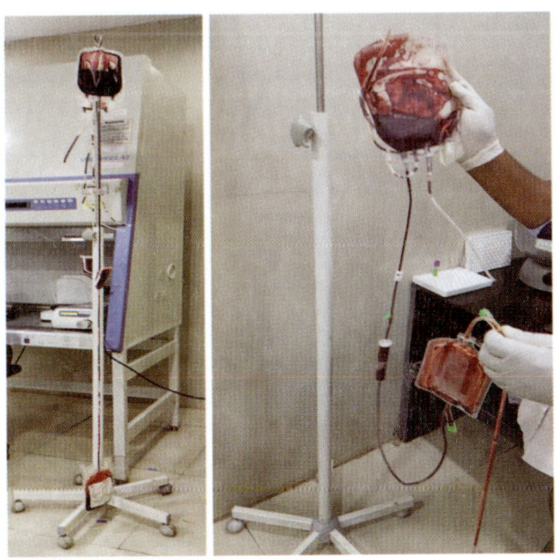

Fig. 6.4: Leukocyte poor packed cell preparation by CRC filter

PREPARATION OF DIFFERENT COMPONENTS IN TOP AND BOTTOM QUADRUPLE BLOOD BAGS

Principle

Same as that of a penta bag. The only difference is the leuko filter is not here and the SAGM is there in the RBC satellite bag.

The quadruple bags contain:

- Mother bag: Contains CPD solution
- Plasma bag
- PRBC bag (with SAGM-2)
- Platelet bag

The mother bag is attached to the plasma and platelet bag at the top, while the SAGM-2 bag is attached to the bottom of the mother bag (Fig. 6.5).

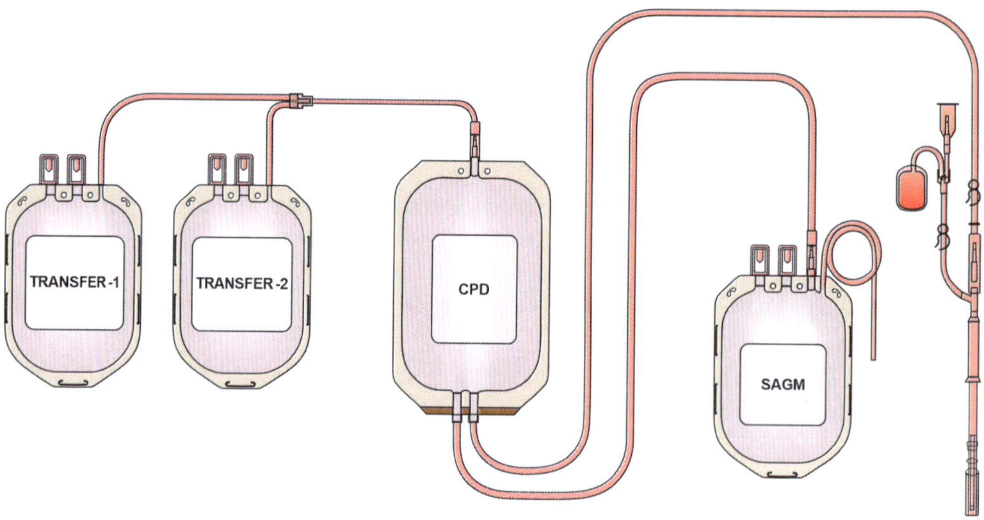

Fig. 6.5: Top and bottom quadruple bags

Step 1

Centrifugation Technique

Same as the above.

Separation Technique

- Open the chamber window of the automatic component extractor machine and place the mother bag inside the chamber on a hanger. Do not disturb the layers, while placing the mother bag on a hanger without any turbulence. Then close the window.
- Hang the mother bag and the satellite bag with SAGM-2 on the hanger which is on the right side in the horizontal direction at 180° angle according to the manual instruction.
- Hang the empty satellite bag (PPP collection) on the hanger over the mother bag according to the manual instruction.

- Hang the platelet satellite bag on a hanger over the red blood cells transfer bag according to the manual instruction.
- Place satellite bag tubing inside the channel clump cum sealer according to the manual instruction (Fig. 6.6).

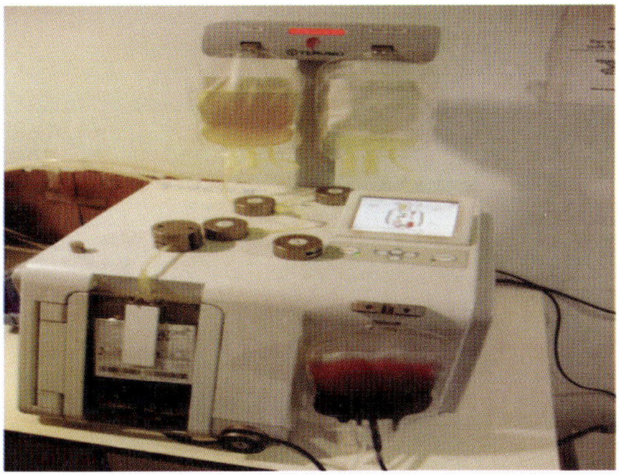

Fig. 6.6: Preparation of different components in top and bottom quadruple bags

- Respective satellite bags should hang on the hanger according to the manufacturer's manual instruction, because these positions may differ from machine to machine.
- Before starting the machine, check thoroughly the automated component separation extractor as per manual instruction.
- Select the program as per manual instruction.
- Immediately break the mother bag and red cells transfer the satellite bag manually and start the machine.
- Now initially 5–10 ml top layer plasma comes from the mother bag automatically upwards direction through connecting tube and is stored in a platelet collection satellite bag. This plasma will help to remove red cells present in click tips. By doing this we get plasma without contamination and it is used for buffy-coat dilution or tubing clean during platelets concentration preparation.

  Then the machine will stop automatically as per programming.
- Remaining top layer plasma comes automatically from the mother bag is transferred in an empty satellite (PPP) collection bag through the connecting tube while the red cell layer is transferred into the bottom bag (SAGM-2) present in the downward position through the connecting tube.
- After completion of the plasma collection and red cells collection, the buffy-coat remains in the mother bag. A few ml of plasma will drip down from the PPP collection satellite bag and mix automatically with the buffy-coat.
- Manually clamp the tubing of platelet collection satellite bag.
- Plasma bag (PPP) and red cells bag will be sealed automatically.
- ACS system will stop automatically as per programming.
- Volume of plasma level varies and it depends on the donor's packed cell volume.
- Detach the plasma (PPP) bag from the remaining satellite bags.
- Detach the red cells bag from mother bag.

- Now the buffy-coat bag is already attached to the platelet collection bag.
- Store platelet-poor plasma (PPP) bag at –80°C or –40°C deep freeze for one year and this plasma is termed as fresh frozen plasma (FFP).
- Store the SAGM-2 blood bag at 2°–6°C in the blood bank refrigerator for 42 days.

PLATELETS CONCENTRATION PREPARATION BY BUFFY-COAT METHOD

Step II

Same as described for the penta bags.

- Steps and procedures of blood component preparation may differ from machine to machine (automated) and it should follow the manufacturer's manual instruction and blood centre SOP.

PREPARATION OF DIFFERENT COMPONENTS IN TOP AND TOP QUADRUPLE BLOOD BAGS (450 ml/350 ml)

Principle

All the bags are connected at their top (Fig. 6.7).

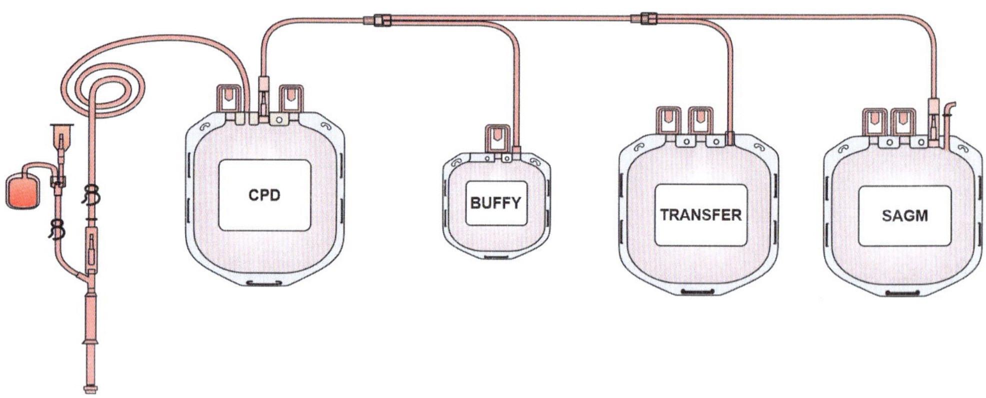

Fig. 6.7: Top and top quadruple blood bags

Step 1

Centrifugation Technique

Same as that of the above-described method.

- Hard spin results in three layers inside the mother bag. The top layer is plasma, (platelets poor plasma, PPP). The middle layer contains buffy coat and the bottom layer contains the red cell concentration.

Separation Technique

- Open the chamber window of the automatic component separation extractor system and place the mother bag inside the chamber on the hanger. Do not disturb while placing the mother bag on the hanger without any turbulence. Then close the window.
- Hang buffy-coat 100 ml transfer satellite bag on a hanger right side in a horizontal direction at 180° angle according to the manual instruction (Fig. 6.8).
- Hang an empty satellite bag (PPP collection) on the hanger over the mother bag according to the manual instruction.

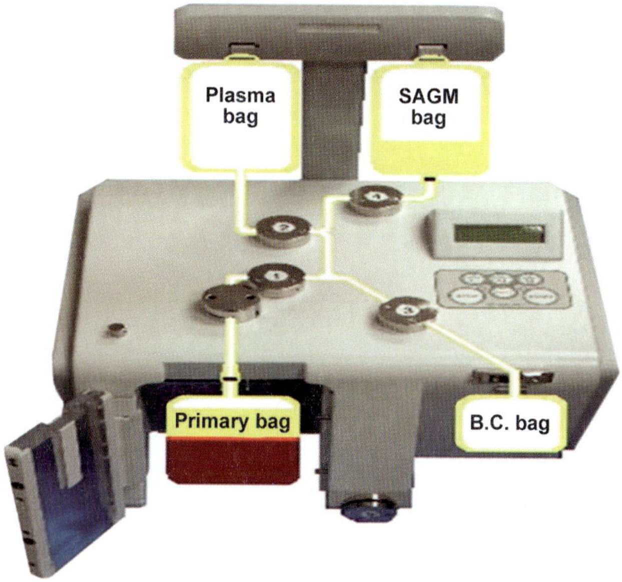

Fig. 6.8: Blood components separation technique by automachine

- Hang the SAGM-2 preservative satellite bag on the hanger over the buffy-coat transfer bag according to the manual instruction.
- Place satellite tubing inside the channel clump cum sealer according to the manual instruction.
- Before starting, check thoroughly the automated component separation machine as per manual instruction.
- Select the program as per manual instruction.
- Immediately break the mother bag and SAGM-2 preservative bag by manually and start the machine.
- Now initially 5–10 ml top layer plasma comes from the mother bag automatically through connecting tubes in an upward direction and mix with the SAGM-2 preservative bag. This plasma will help to remove red cells present in click tips which prevent red cell contamination of plasma.
- Remaining top layer plasma comes automatically into the PPP collection bag through connecting tubes in an upward direction.

  After the complete collection of plasma, the machine stops automatically as per programming.
- Buffy-coat layer with a few ml of red cells automatically transfer to the small 100 ml of buffy-coat collection bag and stops automatically as per programming.
- The buffy-coat bag will be diluted with a few ml of plasma which comes from the PPP collection bag and mix automatically.
- SAGM-2 preservative with the remaining few ml of plasma is transferred to the mother bag automatically and it gets mixed with red cells.
- PPP bag and red cells with SAGM-2 preservative bag should seal automatically and detach from remaining satellite bags.

- Manually clamp the tubing that connects the empty preservative satellite bag with the buffy-coat bag.
- The machine will then stop automatically as per programming.
- Volume of plasma level varies and it depends on the donor's packed cell volume level.
- Store platelet poor plasma bag (PPP) at –80°C or –40°C deep freeze for one year and it is used as FFP.

SAGM-2 preservative blood bag is stored at 2–6°C in the blood bank refrigerator for 42 days.

Step II

Platelets Concentration Preparation by Buffy-coat Method

Same as that of the buffy-coat method platelet preparation in a penta bag/quadruple bag (top-and-bottom).

- Steps and procedures of blood component preparation may differ from machine to machine (automated) and it should follow the manufacturer's manual instruction and blood centre SOP.

Advantages of buffy-coat method for platelets concentration preparation:

1. Initial "hard spin" removes more plasma from the red blood cells and the volume of platelets poor plasma (PPP) is more.
   a. It ensures a better yield of cryoprecipitate (factors V and VIII).
   b. It reduces the incidence of allergic and anaphylactic reactions.
2. The buffy-coat method is a method of leukoreduction (up to one log reduction of leukocytes)
3. The buffy-coat method results in better yield platelets concentration averaging between 6×10^{10} and 9×10^{10} without any possibilities of red cell contamination.

Automated Whole Blood Processor

The automated whole-blood processing machine incorporates the work of both the refrigerated centrifuge and the automated component extractor. It centrifuges the whole blood and creates 3 layers of plasma, a buffy-coat, and the red cell. And simultaneously separates the plasma and red cells along with transferring the buffy-coat into a small transfer bag. Then manually, we have to pool the buffy-coats (4–6 units) and then again centrifuge to separate the platelet (Fig. 6.9).

The advantages of whole blood automation that are claimed by the manufacturer are as follows:

- Productivity:
  - The platelet yield index feature can help you create more pools of platelets from your daily collections of whole blood.
  - One shift and four automatic devices can process approximately 70,000 units of whole blood annually.
- Compliance:
  - Automatically records processing steps
- Efficiency:
  - Reduces the need for resources, including staff time, equipment, space, standard operating procedures (SOPs), and training

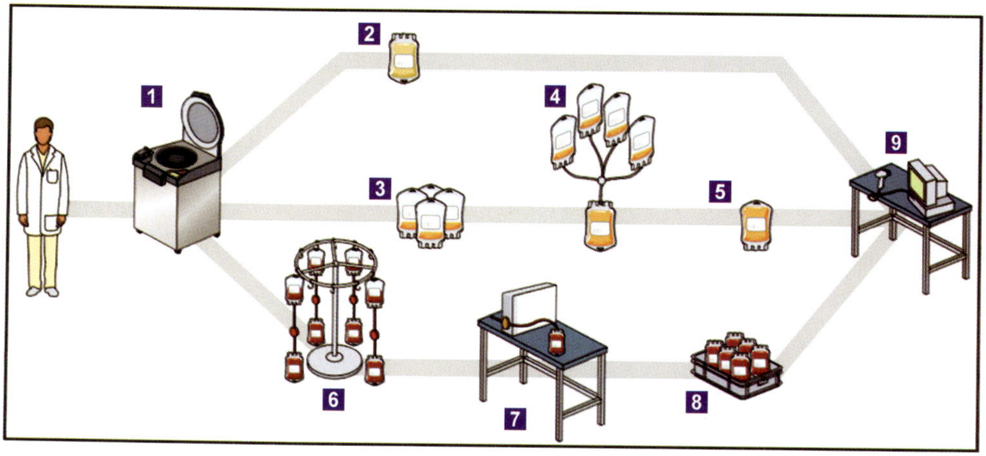

Fig. 6.9: Automated whole-blood processing steps

- In a single run, the system integrates the functions of centrifugation, sedimentation, separation, and sealing of four WB units, resulting in multiple blood components
- Quality:
  - Creates consistent products, using fixed-bucket technology and integrated processing steps
  - Allows for estimating/predicting the platelet yield of platelet pools
  - Plasma is automatically leuko reduced

IMPORTANT INSTRUCTIONS

The automated blood component extractors of different manufacturers or updated versions of the same manufacturer may differ in the positioning of the mother bag and satellite bag, but the ultimate target is to enhance the purity of the blood component by a sharp detection of layers with the help of an intelligent interaction of flow regulator and optical sensors.

DO PRACTICE

1. Ensure a clear detector plate for efficient functioning.
2. Always ensure no moisture outside the tubes.
3. Ensure proper insertion of tubes through clamps and flow regulator.
4. The primary bag (mother bag) has to be placed with the label side visible (in the front position).

DON'T PRACTICE

1. Never use spirit to clean the detector plate. Use soap solution if necessary.
2. Please donot disturb the bags on scales during process. System continuously checking these weights for its functioning.
3. Never apply more force to weighing scales while placing the bags since they are very sensitive.
4. No label should be adhered on the backside of the primary bag (mother bag); sensor plate may not detect the layers.

Chapter 7

Blood Components Therapy

Whole blood is collected as a single unit where with storage platelets are not viable and labile coagulation factors are deficient. Whereas three different components like PRBC, RDP, and FFP can be prepared from a single unit of whole blood and will be helpful to treat three different types of patients with anemia, thrombocytopenia, or coagulopathy. Hence, component therapy is targeted care for patients, and a method of proper resource utilization.

RED BLOOD CELL TRANSFUSION

In patients with anemia, the physiologic compensatory mechanisms are inadequate to maintain normal tissue oxygenation. So, red blood cells (RBCs) are transfused to increase oxygen-carrying capacity in patients with traumatic hemorrhage. But for patients with compensatory anemia like iron deficiency anemia, RBC transfusion is unnecessary.

INDICATIONS

1. Restricted transfusion: Hb <7 gm/dl.
2. Hb <8 gm/dl in patients with cardiac disease.
3. Thalassemia patient's Hb should be maintained at 9–10 gm/dl.

Selection of RBC Unit

- ABO-compatible red cell unit is selected for the patients to avoid acute hemolytic transfusion reaction by the ABO isoagglutinin.
- O group red cell unit is selected as a universal donor for patients in different clinical scenarios as it lacks both "A" and "B" antigens.
- The donor unit selection for different ABO blood group patients is given in Table 7.1.

Table 7.1: ABO group selection (donor) for PRBC transfusion in different ABO group patients

Recipient blood group	*1st choice donor unit*	*2nd choice donor unit*
A	A	O
B	B	O
O	O	A2
AB	AB	A or B or O
Bombay	Bombay	
Rh-positive	Rh-positive	Rh-negative
Rh-negative	Rh-negative	Rh-positive

Rh-negative patients can receive a Rh-positive unit in an emergency (male, old female) but with the consent of the patient and the treating physician.

If a patient is RhD weak positive, it is advisable to choose an Rh-negative donor unit for this patient to avoid the development of anti-D alloimmunization.

PRE-TRANSFUSION TESTING

Pre-transfusion testing basically includes blood grouping and crossmatching. Pretransfusion testing is of three types depending on the type of request (Flowchart 7.1):

1. **Immediate spin crossmatch:** Group specific blood unit is issued by immediate spin crossmatch (15–30 min), DHTR is not ruled out.
2. **Type and screen:** Blood grouping and antibody screening is performed, so that group specific blood unit can be issued without crossmatch if antibody screening is negative. If antibody screening is positive, then antigen negative unit is searched

Flowchart 7.1: The workflow for pre-transfusion testing

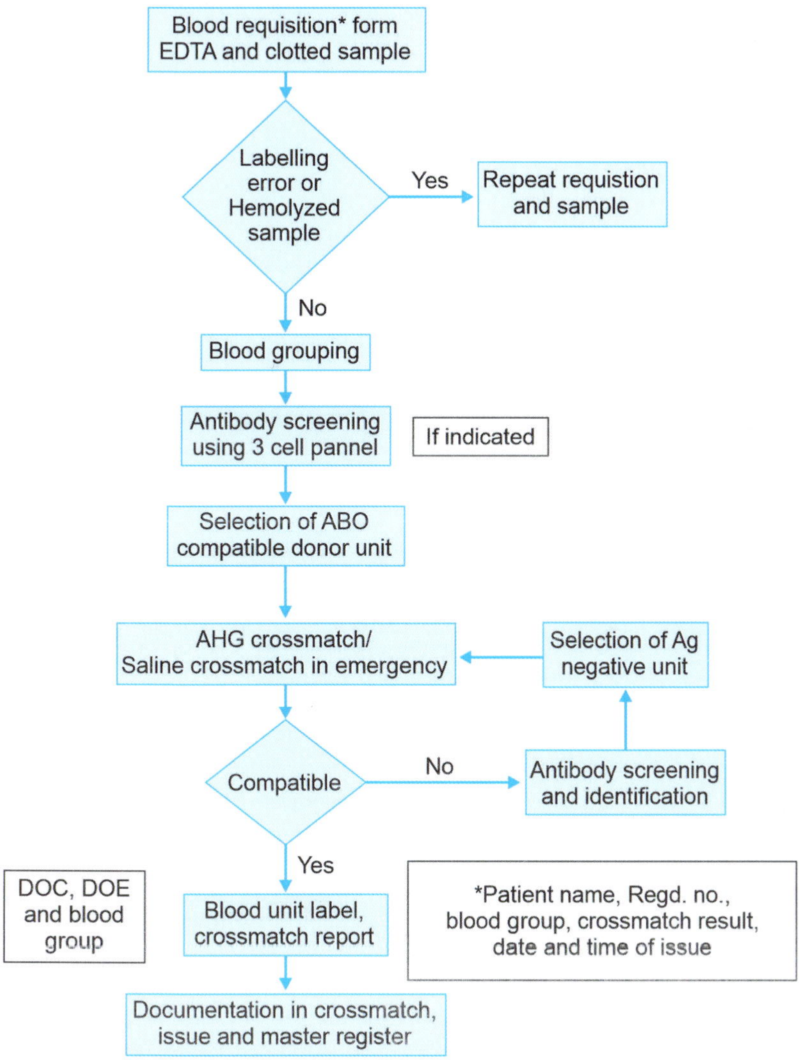

and crossmatched. Antibody screening and extended phenotype are performed in multi-transfused patients to avoid delayed hemolytic transfusion reactions.

3. **Type and crossmatch:** Blood grouping and crossmatching is done for all routine cases where group specific blood unit is crossmatched. It minimises the risk of delayed hemolytic transfusion reactions.

The detailed process of pre-transfusion testing is given in Flowchart 7.1.

Fresh Frozen Plasma/Cryoprecipitate Transfusion

Prophylactic plasma transfusion prior to any invasive procedure to reduce the risk of bleeding is still debatable. Transfusion of plasma is indicated to treat bleeding in various conditions.

INDICATION

1. Patients with multiple coagulation factor deficiencies (e.g. liver disease, DIC).
2. Patients with specific plasma-protein deficiencies (e.g. factor V deficiency) for which a licensed coagulation factor concentrate is not available.
3. Replacement fluid in therapeutic plasma exchange (TTP, HUS, GBS, myasthenia gravis, etc.)
4. Vitamin K antagonist reversal.

Cryoprecipitate

1. Fibrinogen replacement for acquired hypofibrinogenemic conditions such as liver transplantation and postpartum hemorrhage.
2. Congenital hypofibrinogenemia, dysfibrinogenemia, and von Willebrand disease.
3. Congenital factor XIII deficiency.
4. A low fibrinogen concentration among women with postpartum hemorrhage.

Plasma, cryoprecipitate, and fibrinogen concentrate are all sources of fibrinogen. However, the volume of plasma needed is considerably larger than that of cryoprecipitate to achieve the same replacement dose of fibrinogen (e.g. 300–400 mg of fibrinogen can be replaced with 250 ml of plasma or with only 10–15 ml of cryoprecipitate).

Table 7.2: ABO group selection (donor) for FFP transfusion

Recipient blood group	*1st choice donor unit*	*2nd choice donor unit*
A	A	AB
B	B	AB
O	O	AB
AB	AB	

- Same ABO group FFP is selected for transfusion and AB group plasma is the 2nd choice (Table 7.2). There is no such difference in Rh-positive and negative as plasma does not contain Rh antigens. Rh-negative patients can safely be transfused with Rh-positive plasma. Many blood centres also do not mark Rh positive or negative on the plasma bag.
- Cryoprecipitate of any group is issued to the patients, and 4–6 units of cryoprecipitate can also be pooled to issue a patient.

Steps to Issue FFP

- The blood group of the patients should be confirmed and so also the blood group of plasma units.
- Minor crossmatch may be required in newborn babies. Crossmatching is not required routinely. Only group-specific FFP is issued
- Before thawing FFP components, switch on the plasma thawing bath and maintain it at 37°C temperature.
- FFP is thawed in circulating thawing bath at 37°C which usually takes 15–20 minutes and it should not be thawed at room temperature or running tap water.
- The entry ports must be protected so that water cannot contaminate the units.
- Only approved plasma thawing bath maintaining temperature at 37°C should be used to thaw FFPs.
- In the case of pediatric patients, a transfer bag should be used to separate the required volume of FFP from the primary FFP bag using a sterile connecting device. So that a single-unit plasma can be used for a patient for multiple times and hence reduce the number of donor exposure to the patient and so also decrease the wastage of plasma.
- After thawing, issue FFP component product immediately specially for correction of unstable clotting factors. If the issue is delayed, keep it at 4°C and should be used within 24 hours. It cannot be refrozen after thawing.
- The details of FFP should be documented on the issue register, master register and also on the label.

Platelet Transfusion

Platelet transfusions are often administered prophylactically prior to any surgical procedures to reduce the bleeding risk in patients with quantitative or qualitative platelet deficiencies. In a bleeding patient of thrombocytopenia, platelet concentrate is transfused therapeutically.

INDICATIONS

Prophylactic

1. Central venous catheter (TPC $<25 \times 10^9/L$)
2. Lumbar punctures ($<40 \times 10^9/L$) and epidural anesthesia ($<80 \times 10^9/L$)
3. Liver biopsy ($<25 \times 10^9/L$)
4. Major surgery ($<50 \times 10^9/L$), neurosurgery ($<100 \times 10^9/L$)

Therapeutic

1. Major bleeding and thrombocytopenia or massive hemorrhage:	$50–75 \times 10^9/L$
2. Massive transfusion and multiple trauma or TBI:	$75–100 \times 10^9/L$
3. Surgery	$50–100 \times 10^9/L$
4. DIC	$50 \times 10^9/L$
5. DIC in neonates	$100 \times 10^9/L$
6. Intracerebral bleeding	$100 \times 10^9/L$
7. Platelet function defects	No threshold

PLATELET UNIT SELECTION

Table 7.3: ABO group selection (donor) for platelet transfusion

Recipient blood group	*1st choice donor unit*	*2nd choice donor unit*	*3rd choice donor unit*
A	A	AB	O
B	B	AB	O
O	O	A2, AB	
AB	AB	A	B
Rh-positive	Rh-positive	Rh-negative	
Rh-negative	Rh-negative	Rh-positive	

- Any group platelet concentrate (RDP) can be issued to a patient with the consent of the patient and treating physician. ABO identical platelet is preferred for better platelet increment (percentage platelet recovery or corrected count increment). In the A2 blood group donors, the "A" antigen expression is decreased on platelets and therefore preferred for transfusing O or B group patients (Table 7.3).
- Rh-negative patients may be transfused with Rh-positive platelet which doesnot have red cell contamination. Even 7–10 units of Rh positive platelet may also be transfused safely to Rh negative patient under RhIG prophylaxis.

Steps to Issue RDP

- Blood group of the patient and the platelet concentrate should be confirmed prior to issue, and ABO identical platelet transfusion is preferred.
- Platelet conc. should be stored in a platelet agitator-cum-incubator.
- Never store RDP in a domestic refrigerator.
- RDP transfusion should be completed within 30 minutes of issue.
- The details of RDP should be documented on the issue register, master register, and also on the label.

Note: Routinely platelet crossmatching is not performed, but in case of immunological platelet refractoriness, platelet crossmatching is required. Very few centers in India, have the facility for platelet crossmatch. Platelet refractoriness is defined as the clinical condition where the patient does not achieve the anticipated platelet increment following adequate dose of platelet conc. at two instances.

TRANSFUSION RATE AND DURATION OF DIFFERENT BLOOD COMPONENTS

- All the blood components should be transfused through a blood transfusion set with a filter of size 170 microns.
- Correct patient identification and proper blood transfusion note is essential prior to transfusion.
- Take blood transfusion consent from the patient and make him understand the risks and benefits of blood transfusion and the alternatives.
- Post-transfusion, a "no transfusion reaction" or a "utilization certificate" should be produced for the transfusion service. If any transfusion reaction occurs, it should be informed to the blood centre.
- The rate of transfusion of different blood components is given in Table 7.4 and Fig. 7.2.

Table 7.4: Transfusion rate for different blood components

Blood component	*Suggested adult flow rate*		*Remark*
	First 15 min	*After 15 min*	
PRBC	1–2 ml/min 60–120 ml/hour	As rapidly as tolerated approx. 4 ml/min or 240 ml/hr	Should be finished within 4 hours or 2–3 hours in a hemodynamically stable patient
FFP	2–5 ml/min 120–300 ml/hour	As tolerated 300 ml/hour	20–30 min required for thawing
RDP	2–5 ml/min 120–300 ml/hour	As tolerated 300 ml/hour	For patients at risk of fluid overload, a slower rate is required (1 ml/min)
Cryoprecipitate	As rapidly as tolerated		

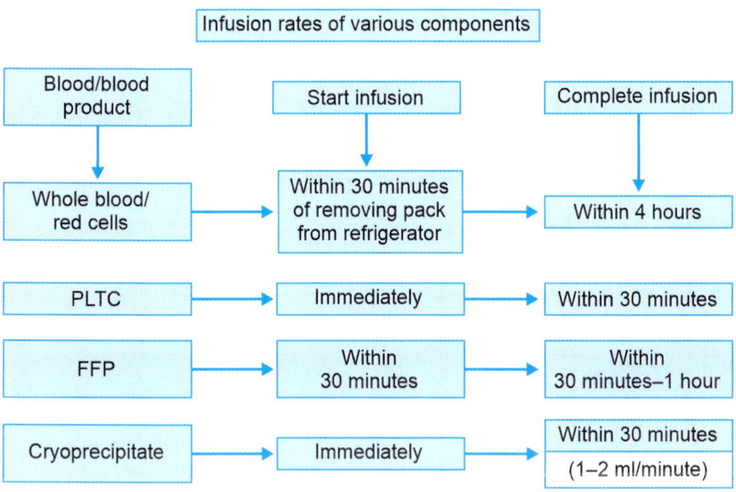

Fig. 7.2: Starting and completion timing of different blood components

Chapter 8

Quality Control

The good quality of blood components depends upon various factors like:

- **Selection of donor:** Healthy, regular donor.
- **Quality of the container and anticoagulant preservative solution:** 450 ml blood bag gives better yield for platelet and plasma.
- **Phlebotomy:** A perfect phlebotomy results in free flow of blood, and hence better platelet yield than blood unit of a slow flow collection.
- **The technique of component preparation:** Buffy coat method gives one log reduction in leukocytes and hence risk of FNHTR is less.
- **SOP:** Adherence to SOP will result good quality of component.
- **Storage temperature:** Proper storage temperature and space is needed for good quality platelet and other components.
- **Preparation duration:** Blood components should be prepared and stored within 6 hours of collection, to preserve the labile coagulation factors.
- **Training of technicians:** A trained technician is an essentiality of good quality assurance.
- **Automation:** Automation has the advantage of better productivity, yield and efficiency.

For quality control of various blood components (Tables 8.1 to 8.9), either 1% of the total collection per month or 4 units per month, whichever is greater, should be tested. Out of

Table 8.1: Quality control of whole blood

Parameters	*Quality requirement*	*Frequency of QC*
Appearance	No hemolysis No turbidity No visible clot No frothy appearance	All units
Volume	350/450 ml ±10%	1% of all units or 4 units per month whichever is maximum
Anticoagulants*	49/63 ml	
PCV (Hct)	30 to 40%	
Sterility	By culture	

Note: *Volume of anticoagulant should be proportionate to the volume of blood. 14 ml of CPD/CPDA-1 anticoagulant solutions is required for 100 ml of blood.
***Drugs** controller general India, National Blood Transfusion Council.

the total tested units, ≥75% of blood components should fulfill the quality requirements. All blood component units should be non-reactive for HIV 1 and 2, HBV, HCV, malaria, and syphilis.

There are different types of blood bag with different volume of collection; like single bag, double bag, triple bag, or quadruple bag with 350 ml or 450 ml volume.

The single bags are mostly 350 ml and whole blood is collected.

- **Visual inspection:** Check for hemolysis, turbidity, or clot.
- **Volume:** Use weighing balance, note the volume.

Vol. (ml) = Weight of blood bag (gm)—weight of empty bag (gm).

- One bag from each new lot should be measured for the volume of anticoagulant and sent for culture.
- **PCV:** Measure the HCT by CBC (hematology analyzer).
- **Sterility:** Send blood bags to the microbiology department for sterility testing.

Table 8.2: QC of red cell Concentration without an additive solution

Parameters	*Quality requirement*	*Frequency of QC*
Appearance	No hemolysis No turbidity No visible clot No frothy appearance	All units
Volume	250 ± 10% (450 ml) 150 ± 10% (350 ml)	1% of all units or 4 units per month whichever is maximum
PCV (Hct)	65 to 70%	
Sterility	By culture	

Table 8.3: QC of red cell concentration with an additive solution

Parameters	*Quality requirement*	*Frequency of QC*
Appearance	No hemolysis No turbidity No visible clot No frothy appearance	All units
Volume	350 ± 10% (450 ml) 250 ± 10% (350 ml)	1% of all units or 4 units per month whichever is maximum
PCV(Hct)	50 to 60%	
Sterility	By culture	

Table 8.4: QC of modified red cell concentration		
Parameters	*Quality requirement*	*Frequency of QC*
Appearance	No hemolysis No turbidity No visible clot No frothy appearance	All units
Volume	350 ± 10% (450 ml) 250 ± 10% (350 ml)	1% of all units or 4 units per month whichever is maximum
PCV(Hct)	50 to 60%	
Leuko reduced Leukocyte count	Leuko filter: <5 × 10^6 Washed: <5 × 10^6 Buffy coat: <5 × 10^8	
Saline washed PRBC	Plasma removed >99% Red cell loss <20%	

Table 8.5: QC of platelet concentrate by platelet-rich plasma		
Parameters	*Quality requirement*	*Frequency of QC*
Appearance	Swirling present, No visual RBC contamination No discoloration	All units
Volume	50–70 ml	1% of all units or 4 units per month whichever is maximum
Platelet count	3.5 × 10^{10} (350 ml bag) 4.5 × 10^{10} (450 ml bag)	
pH	>6.0 (at the end of the permissible storage period)	
RBC contamination	Traces to 0.5 ml	
WBC count	5.5 × 10^7 to 5.5 × 10^8	
Sterility	By culture	

WBC count by Negeotte chamber

Table 8.6: QC of platelet concentrate by buffy-coat method (450 ml)		
Parameters	*Quality requirement*	*Frequency of QC*
Appearance	Swirling present, No visual RBC contamination No discoloration	All units
Volume	70–90 ml	1% of all units or 4 units per month whichever is maximum
Platelet count	>6 × 10^{10}	
pH	>6.0 (at the end of the permissible storage period)	
RBC contamination	Traces to 0.5 ml	
WBC count	<5.5 × 10^7	
Sterility	By culture	

Table 8.7: QC of SDP (apheresis platelet)		
Parameters	*Quality requirement*	*Frequency of QC*
Appearance	Swirling present, No visual RBC contamination No discoloration	All units
Volume	>200 ml	1% of all units or 4 units per month whichever is maximum
Platelet count	$>3 \times 10^{11}$	
pH	>6.0 (at the end of the permissible storage period)	
RBC contamination	Traces to 0.5 ml	
WBC count	$<5.5 \times 10^{6}$	
Sterility	By culture	

PRECAUTIONS TO BE TAKEN WHILE SAMPLING FOR QUALITY CHECK

1. **Adequate mixing:** Mixing of product and proper stripping of tubing is performed so that the sample taken for QC from the tubing represents the actual product. The tubing of the bag containing the sample may be detached using an electric sealer. It prevents any contamination of the full bag as the total bag then send for culture.
2. **Sampling method:**
   - Samples for Hb/platelets count should be taken into a dry EDTA tube.
   - Sampling methods must be validated to ensure that they produce consistent samples, regardless of the operator.
   - RDP bags are randomly selected and checked for the platelet concentration by standard procedure like platelets count analyzer or platelets counting chamber.

Table 8.8: QC of fresh frozen plasma (FFP)		
Parameters	*Quality requirement*	*Frequency of QC*
Appearance	No icteric, lipemia, or discoloration	All units
Volume	180–220 ml (350 ml bag) 220–300 ml (450 ml bag)	1% of all units or 4 units per month whichever is maximum
Factor VIII	70 IU/bag	
Fibrinogen	200–400 mg	

Table 8.9: QC of cryoprecipitate		
Parameters	*Quality requirement*	*Frequency of QC*
Appearance	Slushy consistency	All units
Volume	15–20 ml	1% of all units or 4 units per month whichever is maximum
Factor VIII	At least 80 IU/bag	
Fibrinogen	At least 150 mg/bag	
Factor XIII	20–30% of original	Occasional
vW factor	40–70% of original	Occasional
Fibronectin	150 mg/bag	Occasional

Items Required for Quality Control of Blood Components

1. **Hematology analyzer (Fig. 8.1):** For complete blood count.
2. **pH meter (Fig. 8.2a and b):** To measure the pH of platelet conc.
3. **pH Tablets:** To calibrate the pH meter, three different value pH tablets/solutions are required, e.g. pH 4, 7, 10 (Fig. 8.2a and b).
4. **Coagulation analyzer (Fig. 8.3):** For QC of FFP/cryoprecipitate.
5. **Weighing scale:** To measure the volume of blood components.
6. **Negeotte chamber (Fig. 8.4):** To calculate the leukocyte count.
7. **Neubauer's chamber (Fig. 8.5):** To calculate the RBC, platelet count.

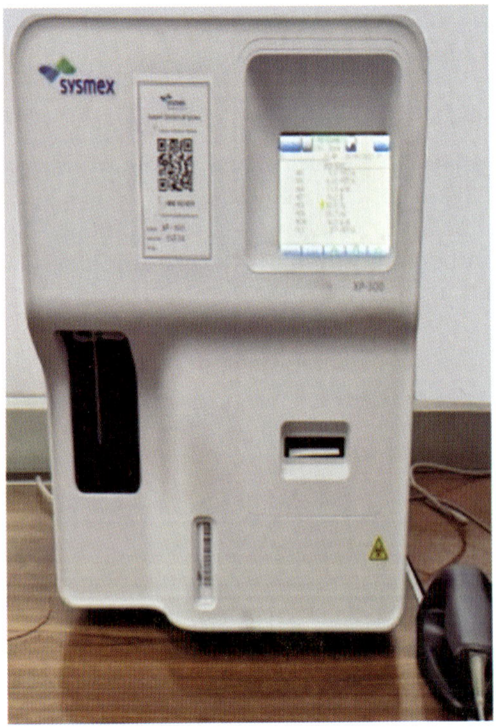

Fig. 8.1: Hematology analyzer

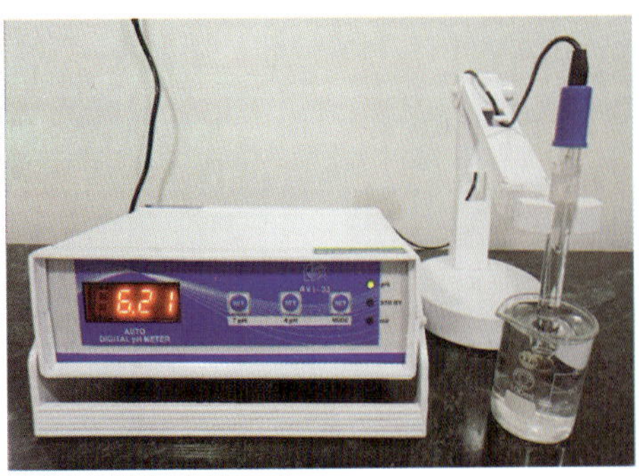

Fig.8.2a: pH meter

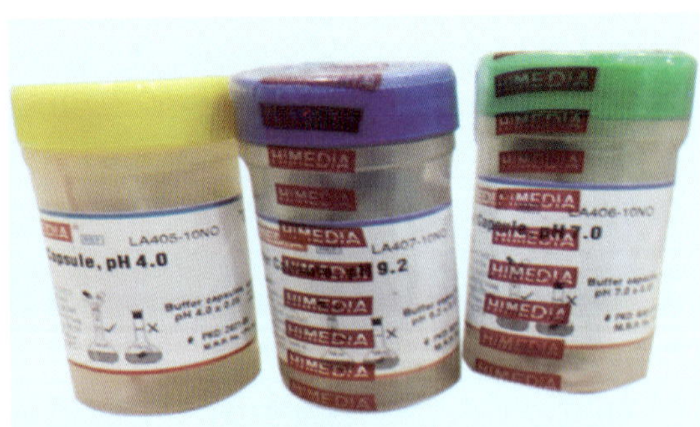

Fig. 8.2b: pH tablets (pH 4.0, 7.0, 10)

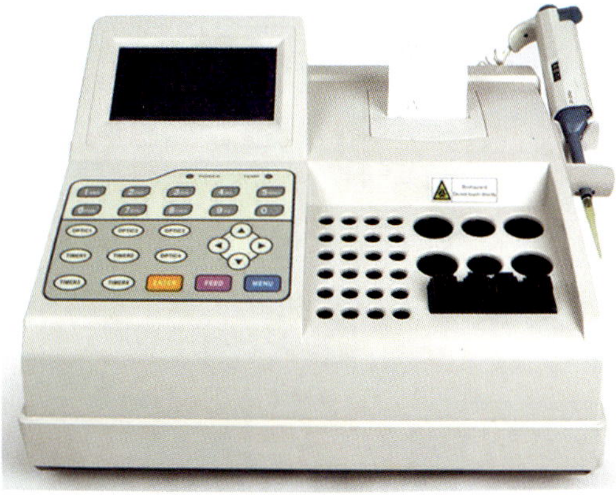

Fig 8.3: Coagulation analyzer

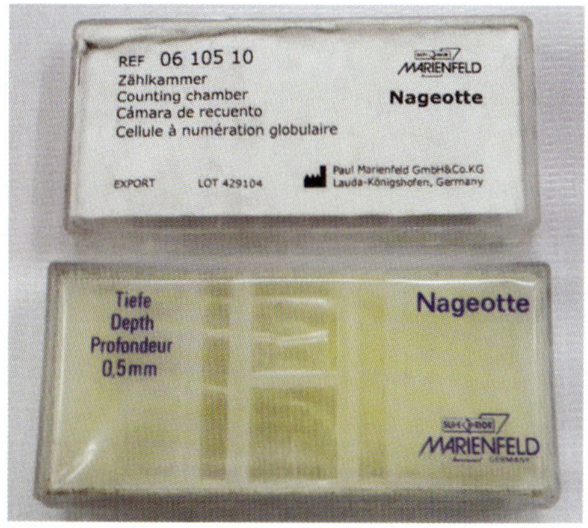

Fig 8.4: Negeotte chamber

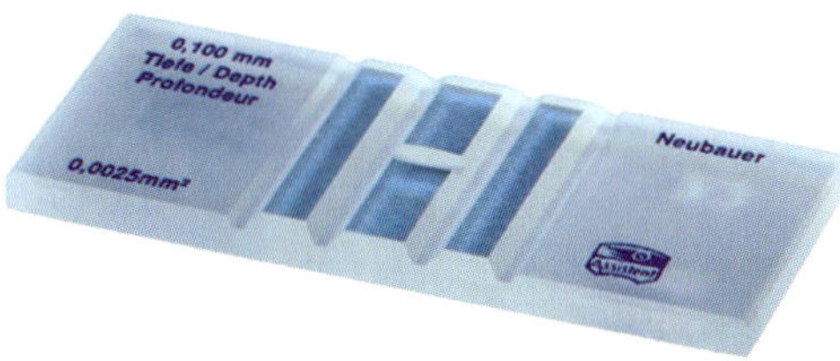

Fig 8.5: Neubauer's chamber

Chapter 9

Biosafety and Biomedical Waste Management

Biosafety in a blood center involves implementing procedures and practices designed to protect both staff and patients from the risks of exposure to bloodborne pathogens and other hazardous materials. Ensuring biosafety is crucial to prevent the transmission of infections, ensure the safety of blood products, and protect the environment and health of all personnel working in the blood center.

Importance of Biosafety in Blood Centre

- **Protecting donors and staff:** Ensures that donors, recipients, and staff are not exposed to infectious agents.
- **Maintaining blood supply integrity:** Ensures blood products are safe for transfusion and contamination-free.
- **Regulatory requirements:** Compliance with regulatory bodies to avoid legal and financial repercussions.

KEY COMPONENTS OF BIOSAFETY IN A BLOOD CENTER

1. Infection Control Protocols

- **Universal precautions:** Treat all blood and blood products as potentially infectious, regardless of the perceived status of the donor.
- **Personal protective equipment (PPE):** Use of gloves, gowns, masks, and eye protection when handling blood products or when there is a risk of exposure.
- **Hand hygiene:** Frequent hand washing with soap and water or using alcohol-based hand sanitizers, especially after removing gloves or handling blood products.

2. Safe Handling of Blood Products, Specimen or Samples, Techniques

- **Proper techniques for collection, component separation and storage:** Using sterile needles and equipment, and ensuring minimal contamination during the collection process, component separation, and storage. All equipment should be handled properly as per the manufacturer's instruction.
- **Sample handling:** Proper handling of sample is essential for the safety of HCW.
- **Transport and storage:** Samples and blood products should be transported and stored under conditions that prevent contamination and maintain their viability.

3. Waste Management

Any waste generated during the diagnosis, treatment, or immunization of human beings or animals or research activities pertaining thereof or in the production or testing of biologicals or health camps is defined as biomedical waste. Healthcare facilities (HCF) generate lots of waste which can transmit infections, particularly HIV, hepatitis B, hepatitis C, to the people who handle it or come in contact with it, if not disposed of properly. All such waste that carries a risk of causing harm to the health of a person or environment is considered infectious and should be managed as per Biomedical Waste Management (BMWM) Rules, 2016.

Most countries, especially developing nations, are facing a grim situation arising out of environmental pollution due to pathological waste generated from rapidly growing healthcare centers. India is no exception to this. It is estimated that there are more than 70,000 hospitals in the country. As per a report by state boards in 2022, about 705 tons/day of biomedical waste was generated during 2021–22 by 3,93,939 HCF. As per BMWM rule 2016, BMW shall be treated and disposed of by a common biomedical waste treatment facility (CBWTF). Around 79% of the HCF utilize the CBWTFs for collection, storage, treatment, and disposal of BMW.

The quantity of BMW is around 10–15% of total waste generated from HCFs. BMW includes soiled materials with blood, secretions of patients, infected parts, biological liquids such as urine, fluid, etc. chemicals, medical supplies, medicines, lab discharge, sharps, metallic implants, glassware, and plastics, etc. These BMWs are grouped into four categories based on the segregation pathway and color code, as follows:

i. Yellow category
ii. Red category
iii. White category
iv. Blue category

Each category includes various types of BMW, which are mentioned in Table 9.1.

Table 9.1: Different category of BMW as per BMWM Guideline 2016

Yellow category	
Human anatomical waste	Human tissues, organs, body parts and fetus below the viability period (as per the Medical Termination of Pregnancy Act 1971, amended from time to time).
Animal anatomical waste	Experimental animal carcasses, body parts, organs, tissues, including the waste generated from animals used in experiments or testing in veterinary hospitals or colleges or animal houses
Soiled waste items	Items contaminated with blood, body fluids like dressings, plaster casts, cotton swabs and bags containing residual or discarded blood and blood components.
Discarded or expired medicine	Pharmaceutical waste like antibiotics, cytotoxic drugs including all items contaminated with cytotoxic drugs along with glass or plastic ampoules, vials, etc.
Chemical [illegible]	[illegible]micals used in production of biological and used or [illegible] disinfectants

(Contd...)

Table 9.1: Different category of BMW as per BMWM Guideline 2016 *(Contd…)*	
Yellow category	
Chemical liquid waste	Liquid waste generated due to the use of chemicals in the production of biological and used or discarded disinfectants, Silver X-ray film developing liquid, discarded Formalin, infected secretions, aspirated body fluids, liquid from laboratories and floor washings, cleaning, house-keeping and disinfecting activities, etc.
Discarded linen, mattresses, beddings contaminated with blood or body fluid, routine mask and gown.	
Microbiology, biotechnology and other clinical laboratory waste (pre-treated)	Microbiology, biotechnology and other clinical laboratory waste: Blood bags, laboratory cultures, stocks or specimens of microorganisms, live or attenuated vaccines, human and animal cell cultures used in research, industrial laboratories, production of biological, residual toxins, dishes and devices used for cultures.
Collection: Collect the waste in yellow-coloured non-chlorinated plastic bags and store in a yellow-coloured container. **Treatment/disposal options:** Incineration or plasma pyrolysis or deep burial*. In the absence of the above facility for soiled waste items, autoclaving or micro-waving/ hydroclaving followed by shredding or mutilation or a combination of sterilization and shredding. Treated waste is to be sent for energy recovery. **Drugs:** All discarded medicines shall be either sent back to the manufacturer or disposed by incineration. **Chemical waste:** Incineration or plasma pyrolysis or encapsulation. **Discarded linen/mattresses:** Non-chlorinated chemical disinfection followed by incineration or plasma pyrolysis or for energy recovery.	
Red category	
Wastes generated from disposable items such as tubing, bottles, intravenous tubes and sets, catheters, urine bags, syringes without needles, vacutainers and gloves.	
Treatment/disposal options: Autoclaving or micro-waving/hydroclaving followed by shredding or mutilation or combination of sterilization and shredding. Treated waste to be sent to registered or authorized recyclers or for energy recovery or plastics to diesel or fuel oil or for road making.	
White category	
Waste Sharps including metal needles, syringes with fixed needles, needles from needle tip cutters or burners, scalpels, blades, or any other contaminated sharp object that may cause punctures and cuts. This includes both used, discarded and contaminated metal sharps.	
Container: Puncture-proof, leak-proof, tamper-proof containers. **Treatment/disposal options:** Autoclaving or dry heat sterilization followed by shredding or mutilation or encapsulation in metal container or cement concrete; combination of shredding cum autoclaving; and sent for final disposal to iron foundries.	
Blue category	
Broken or discarded and contaminated glass including medicine vials and ampoules except those contaminated with cytotoxic wastes.	
Container: Cardboard boxes with blue colored marking. **Treatment/disposal options:** Disinfection (by soaking the [illegible] with detergent and sodium hypochlorite treatment) [illegible] hydroclaving and then send for recycling.	

*Disposal by deep burial is permitte[illegible]

Steps Involved in Bio-medical Waste Management

1. Segregation
2. Collection
3. Pre-treatment
4. Intramural transportation
5. Storage
6. Treatment
7. Disposal

The HCF is responsible for the first five steps, i.e. from segregation to storage of BMW. While CBWTF is responsible for the transportation of the BMW from HCF and treatment and final disposal of the waste. The responsibilities of the HCF for managing the BMW are as follows:

- Segregation at the point of generation by the person who is generating the waste in a designated color-coded bin/container.
- Do not mix the BMW with the general waste.
- Storage time of waste should be as little as possible so that waste storage, transportation, and disposal are done within 48 hours.
- Phase out the use of chlorinated plastic bags (excluding blood bags) and gloves by 27/3/2019.
- No secondary handling or pilferage of waste shall be done at HCF.
- If a CBWTF facility is available at a distance of 75 km from the HCF, bio-medical waste should be treated and disposed only through such CBWTF operator.
- Only laboratory and highly infectious waste shall be pre-treated onsite before sending for final treatment or disposal through a CBWTF operator.
- Provide bar-code labels on all color-coded bags or containers containing segregated bio-medical waste before such waste goes for final disposal through a CBWTF.

BMW Generated at Blood Centre

Area	*BMW*	*Category*	*Treatment/final disposal*
Donor screening area	Swabs	Yellow bag	Incineration
	Lancets	Puncture proof white translucent	Landfill/safe pit
	Hb-cuvette	Red bag	Autoclave shredder
	Gloves (all areas)	Red bag	
Bleeding room/ apheresis	Swabs	Yellow bag	Incineration
	Needle of the bag	Puncture proof white	Landfill/safe pit
	Blood bag tubing without needle, diversion pouch	Autoclave/yellow bag	Incineration
	Syringe without needle	Red bag	Autoclave shredder
	Apheresis kit	Red bag	
	Adhesive tape	Red bag	
	Plasma bag collected in TPE	Autoclave/yellow bag	Incineration

(Contd...)

Area	*BMW*	*Category*	*Treatment/final disposal*
TTI screening lab	Sample tubes	Red bag	Autoclave shredder
	Discarded ELISA plate	Red bag	
	Micro-tips	Red bag	
	Washer waste, chemical reagents, kit controls	Hypochlorite treatment yellow bag	ETP
	Rapid card	Yellow bag	Incineration
	Reactive blood component	Autoclave/yellow bag	Incineration
Component lab	Blood bag tubing with blood, buffy coat, leaked/broken/ruptured blood bag, inline filter	Autoclave/yellow bag	Incineration
Serology lab (IH lab)	Empty glass vials of the antisera/lectin/panel cells/albumin/pasture pipette	Blue	Autoclave/hypochlorite treatment then send for recycle
	Blood bag tubing	Red bag	Autoclave shredder
	Broken test tubes/slide	Blue	Sharp pit
	Micro-tips	Red bag	Autoclave/shredder
	Gel cards	Yellow	Incineration
	Blotting paper/swab	Yellow	Incineration
General waste	Wrappers (blood bag, kit) Wrappers and bottles from refreshment for donors	Black	Landfill, recycle

BMWM at Blood Centre

BMWM in the HCF including the blood centre should be as per the BMWM rule 2016, as follows:

- BMW at blood centre should be segregated as per the category mentioned above at the site of production by the technician/nursing staff/supporting staffs on duty at that laboratory.
- Posters/placards for biomedical waste segregation should be provided in all the wards as well as in waste storage area.
- Adequate number of color coded bins/containers and bags should be available at the point of generation of bio-medical waste (donor complex area, blood group serology lab, TTI screening lab, blood component separation lab, etc.)
- Color coded plastic bags should be in line with the Plastic Waste Management Rules, 2016.
- Collection of BMW should be daily at a fixed time, and general waste collection timing should be different.
- Biomedical waste bags and sharps containers should be filled to no more than three quarters full. Once this level is reached, they should be sealed ready for collection.
- Plastic bags should never be stapled but may be tied or sealed with a plastic tag or tie.
- Replacement bags or containers should be available at each waste-collection location so that full ones can immediately be replaced.

- Biomedical waste bags/containers are required to be provided with bar code labels in accordance with CPCB (central pollution control board) guidelines for "guidelines for barcode system for effective management of biomedical waste".
- Interim storage of biomedical waste is discouraged in the wards/different departments of HCF.
- If waste is needed to be stored on interim basis in the departments it must be stored in the dirty utility/sections.
- In house transportation of biomedical waste from site of waste generation/interim storage to central waste collection centre, within the premises of the hospital must be done in closed trolleys/containers preferably fitted with wheels for easy manoeuvrability.

Preparation of Required Concentration of Hypochlorite Solution and its Utilization in Blood Centre

Sodium hypochlorite is used for disinfecting working surface, frequently touched objects, sterilization of medical equipment (1%), and spill management (5%) at the blood centre. The stock solution (commercially available) is usually of 5% or 4%, which is converted to 1% or 5% as follows:

$$C1V1 = C2V2$$

To prepare, 500 ml 1% sodium hypochlorite solution from 5% solution

$$5\% \times V1 = 1\% \times 500 = 500$$

$$V1 = 500/5 = 100 \text{ ml}$$

So 100 ml 5% sodium hypochlorite is mixed with 400 ml (500 minus 100 ml) distilled water to prepare 1% sod. hypochlorite solution.

To prepare 1000 ml 1% sodium hypochlorite solution from 4% solution

250 ml of 4% sodium hypochlorite is mixed with 750 ml (1000 minus 250 ml) distilled water to prepare 1000 ml of 1% sodium hypochlorite solution.

Many a times stock solution (commercially available) is not available in the department or HCF, then 5% sodium hypochlorite solution can be prepared by adding 170 gm bleaching powder in one liter of water (considering 30% chlorine in bleaching powder, to get 5 gm chlorine 16.5 gm of bleaching powder is required; 16.5 × 30% = 5 gm).

Similarly, add 3.5 gm bleaching powder in 100 ml of water to prepare 1% sod—hypochlorite solution.

Disinfection of Work Surfaces

- All work surfaces, walls and floors of the laboratory should be made of impervious washable surfaces.
- The work surfaces should be cleaned and wiped with a disposable wiping sheet dipped in 1% hypochlorite, at every morning and at the end of each duty. It is essential to use thick gloves for cleaning work surfaces.
- It is the responsibility of each lab in-charge to ensure that it is clean and disinfected.
- Laboratories should be kept scrupulously clean and free of bloodstains.

Use of Autoclave in Blood Centre

The discarded blood components (PRBC, FFP, RDP, cryoprecipitate) should be pretreated in autoclave before segregating in yellow color and then handed over to

CBWTF. BMW should be treated in the autoclave (Fig. 9.1) for a temperature of not less than 121°C and pressure of 15 pounds per square inch (PSI) and residence time of not less than 60 minutes. Medical waste shall not be considered as properly treated unless the time, temperature and pressure indicators indicate that the required time, temperature and pressure were reached during the autoclave process. If so, the the process should be repeated till the change in color of the indicator. A chemical is used for validation of the autoclave, in each batch. A biological indicator (geo-bacillus-stearo-thermophilus spores using vials or spore strips) should be used at least once in every week. Records in this regard shall be maintained.

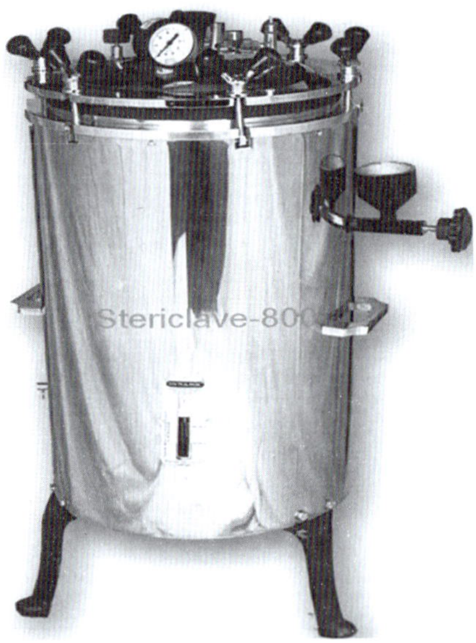

Fig. 9.1: Autoclave (sterilizer)

4. Training and Education

- **Staff training:** Regular training on biosafety protocols, including proper use of PPE, handling of blood products, hand washing and emergency procedures.
- **Continuing education:** Ongoing education to keep staff updated on new risks, emerging pathogens, and best practices in biosafety.

5. Vaccination and Health Monitoring

- **Hepatitis B vaccination:** Vaccination (0,1,6 months) of all staff who may be exposed to blood products. Revaccination should be every 10 years from initial vaccination.
- **Health surveillance:** Regular health checks for staff to monitor for signs of infection or adverse reactions to exposure.

6. Environmental Controls

- **Engineering controls:** Use of safety-engineered devices, like self-sheathing needles, to reduce the risk of accidental injuries.
- **Workplace design:** Blood centers should be designed to minimize the risk of contamination, with separate areas for different activities and appropriate ventilation.

7. Emergency Preparedness

- Exposure incident response
- Spill management.

MANAGEMENT OF NEEDLE STICK INJURY

Following a needle stick injury or mucocutaneous exposure to infectious fluid/blood, all the health workers should be aware of the correction action to deal with the situation immediately and appropriately. After accidental exposure to infectious fluid, the following steps are to be followed:

1. Do not panic, do not place the pricked finger into mouth, do not use antiseptic, iodine, alcohol, bleach, detergent
2. Stay calm
3. Remove gloves, if appropriate
4. Wash exposed site thoroughly:
   a. *For skin:*
      i. Immediately wash the wound and surrounding skin with water and soap and rinse with flowing water or normal saline.
      ii. Mucous exposure: Immediately wash the area, do not use antibiotics/antiseptic
      iii. Do not scrub. Do not use antiseptics
   b. *For eye:* Immediately irrigate the eye thoroughly with running tap water or normal saline (if eye wash station available flush eye) for 15 minutes. Keep the eye open and rotate the eyeballs in all directions to remove contamination from around the eyes.
   c. *For mouth:* Spit out immediately and rinse mouth thoroughly using water or saline. Do not use soap or disinfectant in the mouth.
5. Identify the source:
   a. If source is negative, no need to take postexposure prophylaxis (PEP)
   b. If source is positive for HIV/HBV, or unknown, then take PEP.
6. Reporting to the infection control team/casualty medical officer for management of exposure immediately
7. Risk assessment:
   a. *Mild exposure:* Mucous membrane or non-intact skin with small volume
   b. *Moderate exposure:* Mucous membrane or non-intact skin with large volume or percutaneous superficial exposure, e.g. needle stick injury penetrating gloves
   c. *Severe exposure:* Percutaneous with large volume, e.g. high caliber needle 18G injury, deep wound, transmission of significant volume of blood, etc.
8. PEP
   a. 1st dose of PEP should be administered within 2 hours, but certainly within 72 hours.
   b. Testing of both source and HCW for HIV, HBV, HCV (take consent).
   c. *Testing of HCW:* If previously vaccinated for HBV, then is tested for titer. (10 mIU/ml)

PEP Recommendation for HIV		
Exposure code (EC)	*HIV source code (SC)*	*PEP recommendation*
EC1: Mucous membrane/non-intact Skin: Small volume/few drops short duration	SC1: (HIV positive): Low titer exposure (asymptomatic/ high CD4)	PEP may not be warranted (exposure type does not pose a known risk for HIV transmission)
EC1	SC2: High titer (advanced AIDS, high or low viral load)	Consider basic regimen Negligible risk
EC2: Large volume-major splash/ long duration Percutaneous exposure: Less sever solid needle/superficial scratch	SC1	Recommended basic regimen
EC2	SC2	Recommend expanded regimen. No increase rsssisk for HIV transmission
EC3: Percutaneous exposure: Hollow bore needle, deep injury	SC1 or SC2	Recommend expanded regimen. Increase risk for HIV transmission
Unknown		Basic regimen

Tenofovir 300 mg + Lamivudine 300 mg + Efavirenz 600 mg OD for 28 days

PEP Recommendation for HBV (hepatitis B)			
Exposure		*Source*	
Vaccination/serostatus	HBsAg positive	HBsAg negative	Unknown
Unvaccinated	HBIG single dose Initiate vaccination	Initiate vaccination	Initiate vaccination
Responder (Titer >10 mIU/ml)	No treatment	No treatment	No treatment
Non responder			
After one series of vaccination (3 dose)	HBIG single dose Initiate vaccination	No treatment	HBIG single dose Initiate vaccination
After two series of vaccination (6 dose)	HBIG two dose 1 month apart	No treatment	HBIG single dose Initiate vaccination
Response unknown	Test for anti-HBs If >10: No treatment If <10: HBIG, booster dose vaccine	No treatment	Test for anti-HBs If >10: No treatment If <10: Revaccinate

Managing Spills of Blood and Plasma

- Keep the caution board at the spill area.
- Use PPE (gloves, masks, and protective gown) while handling the spill.
- Put a filter paper sheet or absorbent material over the infected material/blood.

- Pour 5% sodium hypochlorite over and around the absorbent material and leave for 10–15 minutes. (If 1% sodium hypochlorite is used, then contact time should be for 30 minutes)
- Clean the mixture of disinfectant and spilled material with absorbent material using a spatula and contaminated waste container. Discard it into a yellow bin.
- Wipe the surface again with hypochlorite.
- Broken glass/plastic should be swept with a brush and dustpan (do not use hands).
- All spills and accidents are to be reported to the laboratory supervisor.
- Rearrange the spill kit
- Do not use the washing machine to launder mercury contaminated clothing.

8. Regulatory Compliance

- **Adherence to guidelines:** Compliance with local, national, and international guidelines and standards for blood safety and biosafety.
- **Inspections and audits:** Regular inspections and audits to ensure adherence to biosafety protocols and to identify areas for improvement.

Chapter 10

Licensing for Blood Centre and Equipment Management

BLOOD STORAGE CENTRE

Blood storage centres (BSC) are designed to cater the transfusion service to the patients attending first referral units, CHCs, and PHCs or a newly developing hospital/institute. The aim is to make abundant availability of whole human blood or its components to the said hospitals without obtaining a license. However, this exemption is applicable to those centers, which are transfusing blood and/or its components less than 2000 units per annum. However, the licensing authority has laid down regulatory norms for safe storage and the issue of quality blood units. The hospital has to obtain approval from the state drug controller and prior to that consent from the blood centre that has been agreed to be the mother blood centre. The mother blood centre could be a licensed blood centre run by government hospitals/Indian Red Cross/regional blood transfusion centre only. In case the license of the parent blood centre is canceled, the license of the storage centre will also be automatically canceled. The storage centres, however, get affiliated with more than one blood centre to ensure uninterrupted supplies, but separate approval will be required in each case.

REQUIREMENTS

1. **Space:** The area required for setting up a blood storage centre is only 10 square meters, well-lighted, clean, and preferably air-conditioned.

   The map of the BSC should be approved by the superintendent engineer and it should clearly define the situation and flooring area.

2. **Manpower:** One medical officer (doctor, MD-Transfusion Medicine/Pathology) and laboratory technicians are designated for the smooth functioning of the BSc. The MO is responsible for the overall functioning of the BSC. Technicians with blood centre experience are preferred. If the technicians do not have experience in a blood centre previously, then training regarding blood grouping, crossmatching, storage, issue of blood units, management of transfusion reaction, and troubleshooting should be arranged for three days at the mother blood centre or the blood centres at medical colleges, regional blood centres, Indian Red Cross blood centres, or any other well setup, licensed blood centre, provided they have the necessary infrastructure for undertaking training.

3. **Electricity:** Regular 24 hours supply is essential. Provision of backup Generator is required.

A certificate/declaration from the electrical engineer of the hospital is essential.

4. Equipment:

i. *Tabletop centrifuge:* To centrifuge the patient's sample
ii. *Incubator:* To incubate the crossmatch tube (at 37°C)
iii. Gel card centrifuge and incubator
iv. Tube sealer
v. *Blood storage refrigerator:* To store blood units at 4°C
vi. *Reagent refrigerator:* To keep the reagents (antisera) at 4°C
vii. *Deep freezer for ice-packs:* To prepare the ice-packs
viii. *Mobile transport box:* To transport blood units from the mother blood center to BSC at a regulated temperature.
ix. *Microscope:* To check for agglutination which is not visible to the naked eye.

5. Reagents:

i. *Antisera:* Anti-A, anti-B, anti-D (both IgM, and IgG type), anti-AB
ii. *Lectins:* Anti-A1, anti-H
iii. Coombs antisera or antihuman globulin (AHG)
iv. Albumin (6%)
v. LISS (low ionic strength salt solution)
vi. *Gel cards:* Blood grouping gel card, Coomb's card (Coomb's test and crossmatching)

6. Consumables:

i. Test tubes
ii. Pasture pipette
iii. Micropipette
iv. Microtips
v. Glass slide
vi. Test tube racks
vii. Tissue paper
viii. Gloves
ix. Marker pens
x. *Hypochlorite solution (5%):* To disinfect the working surface and the test tubes, sample collecting vacutainers are treated with it.

How to Apply for a Blood Storage Centre?

- The hospital intended to make BSC functional has to apply for the same to the state drug controller with the following application format.
- The applicant shall furnish an undertaking to the licensing authority that the captive consumption of Whole Human Blood or Components shall not be more than 2000 units annually.

Application Format

The State Drugs Controller,

(State name)

Sub: Application for grant of approval for the operation of blood storage centre.

Sir/Madam,

I am submitting herewith the application for a grant of approval for the operation of the blood storage centre at .... (Hospital Name)

1. Details of mother blood centre given consent for the supply of whole human blood/ components:
   a. Name of the health facility: **Licensed blood centre name**
   b. Address:
   c. Letter of consent attached: Yes/No
2. Details of the proposed blood storage centre:
   a. Name of the health facility: ....
   b. Address of the health facility: ....
   c. Name of the superintendent/BMO: ....
   d. Rooms available: Yes/No   Site plan (on butter paper) attached: Yes/No
   e. Equipment available Yes/No   List attached: Yes/No
   f. Medical officer responsible for blood storage centre available: Yes/No

      Qualification and experience certificates enclosed: Yes/No
   g. Lab Technician responsible for blood storage centre available: Yes/No

      Qualification and experience certificates enclosed: Yes/No

You are requested to kindly acknowledge the receipt of application and operation of blood storage centre at ____, as early as possible.

Enclosures(s): as above

Yours sincerely,

(Designation with Seal)

Copy for information & necessary action to:

1. Mother Blood (Bank) Centre (Name)
2. Directorate of Health Services.

- As mentioned in the form, the following attachments are to be submitted along with the application form:
  - Location details/site plan (map attested by the superintendent engineer)
  - List of equipment
  - Details of the medical officer (name, qualification, certificates)
  - Details of the technicians (name and certificates)
  - Consent form from mother blood centre (prototype as follows)

"LETTER OF CONSENT"

To Whom it May Concern

This is to certify that blood centre (Bank) licensed in the premises of M/s ______________ situated at ______________ bearing Lic. No. ______________ Valid up to __________ shall act as mother blood centre (Bank) with respect to the proposed blood storage centre to be set up in the premises of M/s ______________ situated at ______________

Subject to the conditions that Blood Storage Centre complies with below conditions:

1. The capacity consumption of Whole Human Blood or components in the above-said centre shall not be more than 2000 units annually.
2. In the event of a change in the technical staff, the matter shall be reported forthwith to the licensing authority.
3. In the event of a change in the name of the licensed blood centre (mother blood centre) from whom the blood units are being procured, the same shall be intimated to the licensing authority for approval.
4. The centre shall apply for renewal three months prior to the date of expiry of the approval/renewal.
5. The centre shall maintain records and registers including the details of procurement of whole human blood IP/packed red blood cell.
6. The center shall store samples of the blood units received as well as patients' sera for a period of 07 (seven) days from the day of transfusion.

Further, blood units/components shall be supplied after obtaining satisfactory clearance with respect to the following mandatory tests from the blood bank:

a. Blood grouping.
b. Hemoglobin of the donor
c. HIV I and II antibodies
d. Hepatitis B surface antigen
e. Hepatitis C antibody
f. Malarial parasite
g. Syphilis or VDRL

The transportation of blood units shall be the responsibility of the applicant blood storage centre who shall get the same ratified through the approving authority (State Licensing Authority) at the time of accord of necessary approval to run the blood storage centre.

Head
Department of Blood Transfusion/
Medical Officer in-Charge

Storage and Transportations

Cold Chain

It is necessary to maintain the cold chain at all levels, i.e. transportation from the mother centre to the issue of blood unit to the patient. This can be achieved by using mobile transportation boxes which monitor the temperature throughout. During transportation, the blood should be properly packed into cold boxes surrounded by ice packs. Icepacks should not come in direct contact with the blood bags.

Storage

The blood units are kept in a blood bank refrigerator at 4–6°C. The temperature of the blood should be monitored continuously. The storage centre should check the condition of blood on receipt from the mother centre and also during the period of storage.

The responsibility of any problem arising from storage, crossmatching, issue and transfusion will be of the storage centre. Any unit of blood showing hemolysis, turbidity, or change in color should not be taken on stock for transfusion. Due care should be taken to maintain sterility of blood by keeping all storage areas clean.

LICENSING PROCEDURE FOR BLOOD CENTRE

The applicant has to submit the Form 27C and the following documents:

i. Location details/site plan (blueprint attested by the superintendent engineer):

   A minimum area of 100 square meters is required and an additional 50 square meters is required for blood component preparation. For apheresis, an area of 10 square meters is essential.

ii. List of equipment:

   Details of equipment: Date of installation, last date of calibration (certificates)

iii. Details of manpower:

   Medical officer (name, qualification, experience)

   Laboratory technicians (name, DMLT/MLT certificate, experience)

   Nursing officers (name, degree certificate, experience)

   Counselor (name, degree certificate, experience)

iv. List of registers, records, and labels:

   Copy of all registers, forms, and logbooks

   Copy of blood component labels

v. Policy and SOPs

vi. Copy of the payment slip (license fee and inspection fee).

FORM 27 C

Application for the grant/renewal of licence for the operation of a blood bank for processing of whole blood and/or preparation of blood components.

1. I/We .... of M/s. .... here by apply for grant of licence renewal of license number .... dated .... to operate a blood bank for processing of whole blood and/or preparation of blood components on the premises situated at ....

2. Name(s) of the item(s)

   a)

   b)

   c)

3. Names, qualifications and experience of the competent technical staff are as under:

   a) Name(s) of medical officer.

   b) Name(s) of technical supervisor.

   c) Name(s) of registered nurse.

   d) Name(s) of blood bank technician.

4. The premises and plant are ready for inspection/will be ready for inspection on ....

5. A license fee of rupees .... and an inspection fee of rupees .... has been credited to the government under the head of account .... (receipt enclosed).

Date ....

Signature ....

Name and Designation ....

EQUIPMENT MANAGEMENT

- Equipment used in the whole blood collection, component preparation, testing, storage, and issue of blood components shall be maintained in a clean and proper manner.
- So, personnel are in place to facilitate cleaning and maintenance.
- The equipment shall be monitored, standardized, and calibrated on a regularly scheduled basis as described in the standard operating procedures (SOPs).

Selecting an Equipment

It is important to consider the test methodology and the available platforms, before selecting equipment. The selection criteria are as follows:

- **Utilisation index:** Number of hours machine runs per day/maximum number of hours machine can be used per day.
- **Performance characteristics:** Accuracy, precision, sensitivity, specificity
- **Pre-installation requirements:** Space, electric point, plumbing/drainage
- Cost
- Reagent required and supply
- Ease of operation
- Availability of manufacturer support/engineer support
- Warranty

Policy for Selection, Procurement and Installation of an Equipment

1. **Design qualification (specifications: Design, requirement, user specification):** On delivery at the blood centre, equipment is inspected that it is as per the specification.

   A certificate of receipt is generated by the user department and the vendor raises a request for installation.
2. **Installation qualification:** The equipment is installed at the desired place (laboratory) as per the manufacturer's instructions.

   Certificate of installation is handed over to the user department mentioning:
   - Model number, serial number, date of installation
   - Physical verification (checked for damage, physical and functional inspection, internal assembly verification)
   - System configuration check (placed on a flat surface, free space around, if required interface to another equipment)
3. **Operational qualification:** It is a validation protocol that provides documentary verification stating that the equipment is functioning as per the specification supplied by the manufacturer/the pre-approved specification. It includes:
   - Display (commanding menu)
   - Input/output
   - Alram
   - Print function
   - Interface (HIS/LIS)
   - Overall function

4. **Performance qualification:** PQ demonstrates that the equipment performs as expected for its intended use in the processes established by the blood center and that the output meets the center's specifications.

   Responsibility of the lab technician/technical supervisor following installation of the equipment:

   - Post-installation of equipment, the engineer from the manufacturer should train the staff regarding the workflow, daily maintenance, troubleshooting, and precautions to be taken.
   - The technical supervisor/technician should keep all the relevant documents (installation certificate, performance certificate, calibration certificate) in place. He should prepare the working principle (SOP) and related flowcharts of work instruction for ease of work with the help of the transfusion medicine specialist. SOP should be displayed beneath the equipment.
   - The equipment should be labeled properly containing the details as follows:
     - Equipment number (like 2023-BDC-DC-001)
       - 2023—year of installation
       - BDC—blood donation complex (area where the equipment is placed)
       - DC—donor couch
       - 001—equipment number
     - Model no, serial no
     - Date of installation
     - Date of last calibration
     - Due date of calibration
     - Service engineer name and contact details
   - A logbook should be maintained where daily functioning, cleanliness, and breakdown details are recorded.
   - There should be a process in place for calibration and monitoring of the equipment.
   - A process should be in place for preventive maintenance where the engineer from the manufacturer should visit the blood centre and do the necessary preventive maintenance and submit the service report (Table 10.1).
   - For a breakdown of the machine at any instance, the technical supervisor/technician should call customer service and register the complaint. The details should be documented in the logbook and should be followed up till the machine becomes functional.
   - There should be a backup plan or machine during the breakdown of equipment, so as to run the routine work smoothly.
   - Equipment shall operate as per the manufacturer instructor so as to ensure compliance with the official requirements and longevity of the equipment.

Table 10.1: Management of different equipment

S. N.	*Equipment*	*Performance*	*Frequency*	*Calibration frequency*
1	Hemoglobinometer	Standardized against cyanomethemoglobin standard	Each day	As often as necessary
2	Blood collection monitor	Weight the blood bag	Each day	As often as necessary
3	Refrigerated blood bag centrifuge	RPM temperature	Each day of use	As often as necessary
4	Double pan weighing balance	Standardise against a known weight	Each day of use	As often as necessary
5	Plasma thawing bath	Temperature with thermometer	Each day of use	As often as necessary
6	Tabletop centrifuge	RPM	Each day of use	6 monthly
7	Blood bank refrigerator	Temperature with thermometer	Each day of use	6 monthly
8	Platelet agitator-incubator	Temperature	Each day of use	6 monthly
9	Autoclave	Temperature pressure	Each day of use	6 monthly
10	ELISA washer/reader	Negative and positive control run	Each run	6 monthly

Chapter 11

Apheresis Technology and Techniques

Apheresis is derived from the Greek word meaning "to remove". An apheresis machine can be used to isolate the specific blood component that is desired from whole blood. The donor is linked to the machine by a sterilized tubing set referred to as an "apheresis kit". The whole blood is directed into the machine where it undergoes processing. The specific component that is sought after is then gathered in a bag, while the remaining materials are returned to the donor.

Terminology Used for Different Blood Components Separation

1. **Cytapheresis:** Cellular elements are removed.

> ***Example:*** Single donor platelet (plateletpheresis): Platelet concentrate is collected from a healthy donor while returning back red cell and plasma to the donor.

2. **Plasmapheresis:** Plasma is removed.

> ***Example:*** Single donor plasma/convalescent plasma: Plasma is collected from the donor while platelets and red cells are returned to the donor.

Therapeutic apheresis is the removal of red blood cells or plasma. In many disorders, the pathophysiology is due to the excess accumulation of cellular elements of blood or the causal agent (antibody), which is there itself in the plasma.

Therapeutic plasma exchange, red cell exchange, therapeutic cytoreduction, photopheresis, and specific selective adsorption are examples of therapeutic apheresis.

Basic Concepts of Apheresis

Centrifugation, filtration, or combination are the basic principles behind apheresis. *Centrifugation* uses centrifugal force and specific gravity of the cellular and plasma components to separate the elements in the blood. The elements are then removed by siphoning off the desired component or spilling the lighter components over a barrier that retains the heavier components. Effective separation by centrifugation is dependent on the centrifuge g-force, determined by the rotations per minute and rotor radius, and the time that blood is exposed to the centrifugal force.

In some systems, *elutriation* is also used. Two opposing forces—a centrifugal force that pushes heavier elements away from the centrifuge center and a pump withdrawal force that pulls the elements to the centrifuge center—separate based on size rather than specific gravity. This principle is used to separate platelets from leukocytes.

Filtration separates elements based on size, where the filter can be a bundle of hollow fibers with pores in their walls or a membrane surface with pores. The pore size determines what passes through the filter and what is retained. Cascade or double-membrane filtration systems remove pathologic substances from the plasma in two steps, using two filters. The first step involves a primary membrane plasma separator to separate the plasma from the cells and a second step of plasma filtration, with smaller pores to remove proteins, such as immunoglobulins.

Centrifugation, the position of outflow tubing:

The red cells having the highest specific gravity (1.08–1.09), remain in the outer layer of the centrifuge channel (1) and plasma with a specific gravity of 1.02–1.03 is at the innermost layer (3), whereas the middle one is the buffy coat layer (2) (platelet sp gravity 1.03–1.04) (Fig. 11.1). The outflow lines are arranged accordingly, i.e. outflow line for red cells is placed nearer to the outer wall of the channel and the plasma line is on the inner wall.

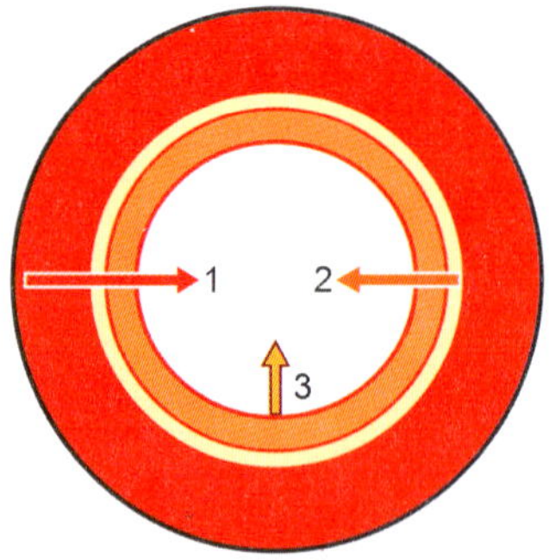

Fig. 11.1: Different layers of blood: (1) Red cell, (2) Buffy coat layer consisting of leukocytes and platelet, (3) Plasma

DIFFERENT TYPES OF APHERESIS MACHINE AND APHERESIS KIT LOADING

1. Trima Accel

Parts of the Apheresis Kit

a. Coil
b. Bag
c. Casset
d. Chanel or filler

Steps of Kit Loading

- Switch on the machine.
- Select the kit loading option on the display screen.
- Open the shield of the plateletpheresis kit.
- Place the bags in their respective hangers.
- Place the cartridge which incorporates most of the tubing with self-loading pump loops, in its designated place as shown in Fig. 11.2.
- Clamp both the needle line and the sample bag line.

- Trima Accel has five pumps and three valves. The pumps are anticoagulant, inlet (draws blood), plasma (moves plasma to a plasma collection bag or return reservoir), platelet (moves platelets to a platelet collection bag or return reservoir; for red cell/ plasma donation, it pumps saline to return reservoir), and return (returns blood). Valves are for the collection of platelets, plasma, or red cells (Fig. 11.3).
- Open the centrifuge chamber using the door latch handle.
- Unlock the filler latch and insert the filler through the loading port.
- Unfold the filler, keep the LRS chamber on the left, and red tubing (RBC line) on the right, and place it on the grove of the filler assembly (Fig. 11.4).
- Put the LRS chamber in its bracket.
- Put the tubing set (collar) in the holder in such a way that there is no twisting, and ensure the locking pin is properly locked.
- Take the loop along the loop arm, keeping the bearings in the lower and upper bearing holders properly.
- Place the tubing set in the upper hex holder properly and rotate the centrifuge to check if any twisting or proper loading is there or not.
- Check the leak detector and close the centrifuge chamber.
- Then put the donor data as demanded by the machine.
- Commands are executed by touching icons on the screen.
- Prick the ACD bag and let a few drops of ACD enter into the tubing till the round valve. Then put the ACD line in the sensor.
- The machine will air-prime the tubing and then prime it with acid.
- Prick the donor, open the sample line, and divert a few drops of blood into the sample pouch, and check the flow whether it is adequate or not.
- Clamp the sample line, open the access line, and follow the command as given by the machine.

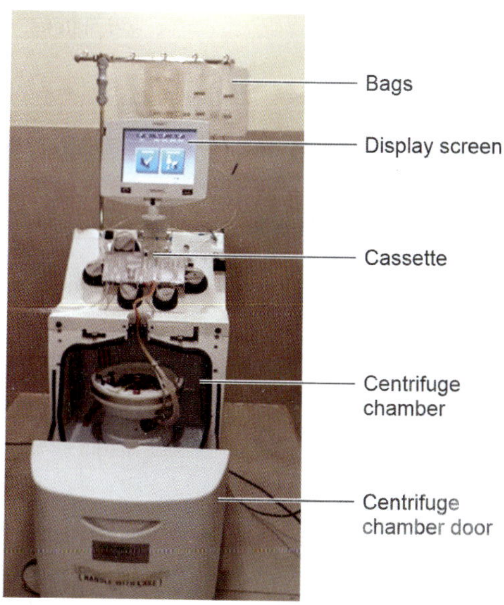

Fig. 11.2: Trima Accel machine and its different outer parts

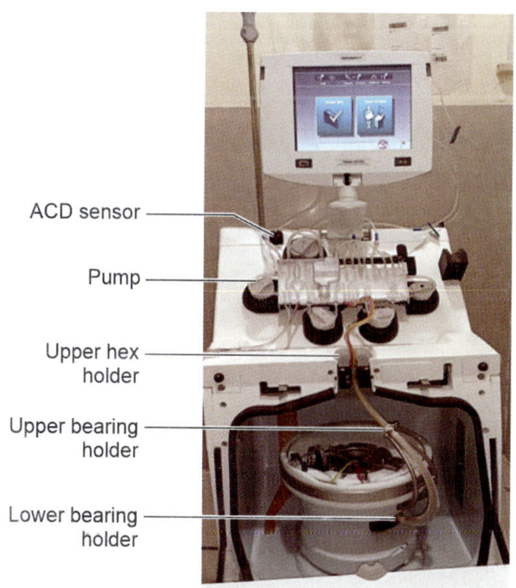

Fig. 11.3: Pumps, valve, and centrifuge chamber of Trima Accel

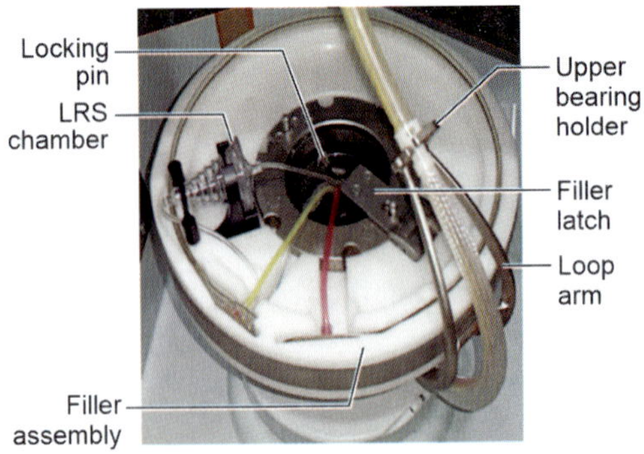

Fig. 11.4: Centrifuge chamber and different parts of the filler assembly

2. Hemonetics MCS+

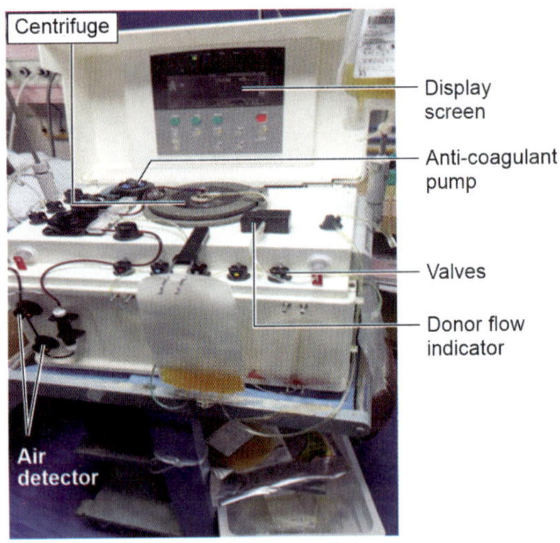

Fig. 11.5: Hemonetics MCS+: Different parts of the machine

3. Amicus

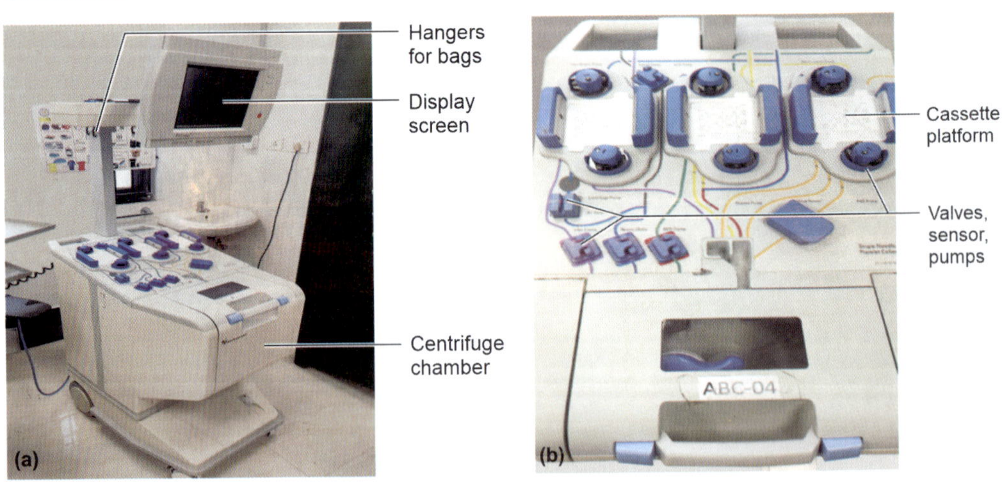

Figs 11.6a and b: Amicus fenwal and its different parts

4. Optia

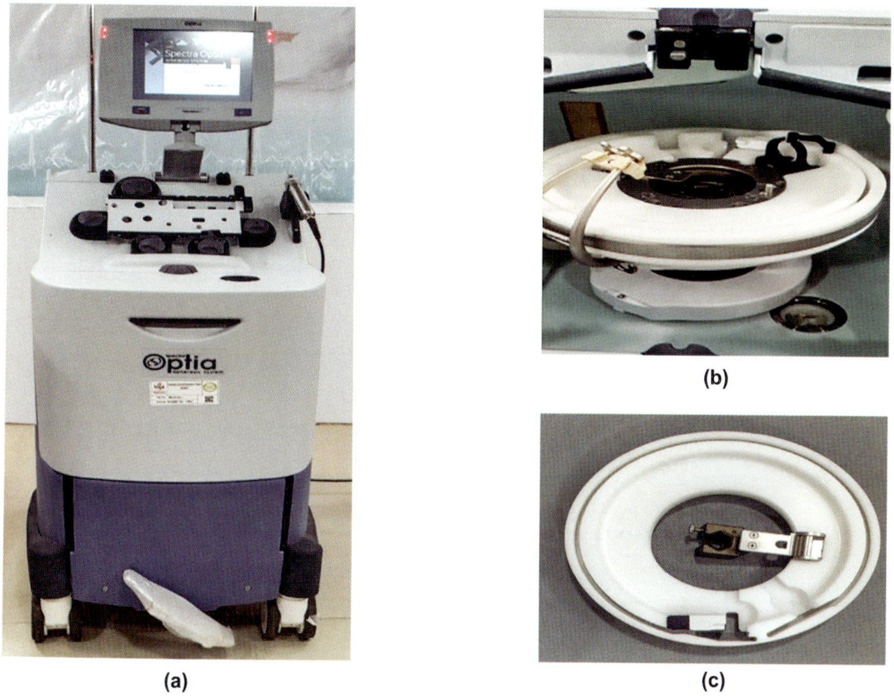

Fig. 11.7a to c: Spectra optia and its two different fillers assembly

5. Fresenius COM.TECH

For the kit loading of this above equipment, please follow the manufacturers' instructions.

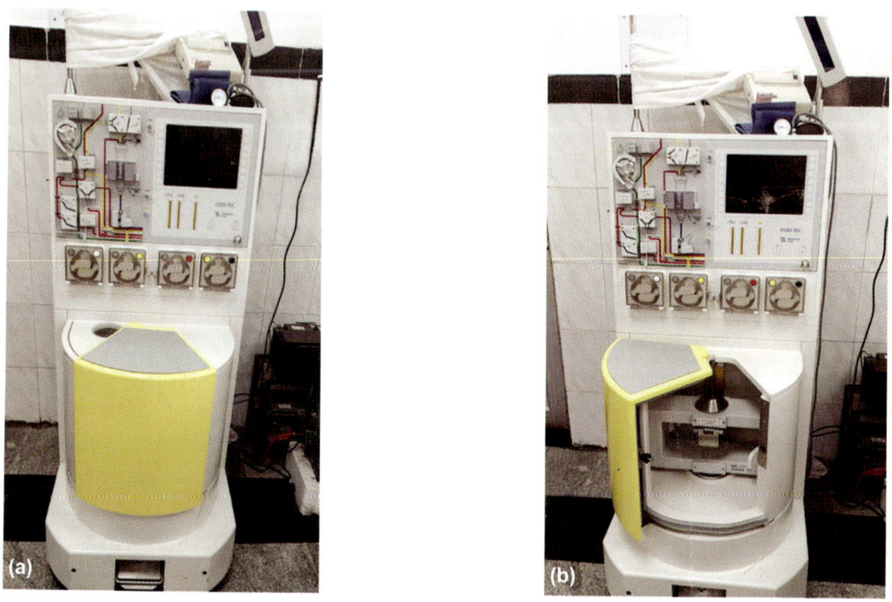

Fig. 11.8a and b: Fresenius Kabi COM.TEC

Donor Selection for Plateletpheresis

The donor selection is similar to whole blood donation, with some different approaches as follows:

a. Height and weight are estimated to calculate the total blood volume, and hence the duration of the procedure as per the yield.
b. Only hemoglobin estimation is done prior to whole blood donation, while complete blood count (CBC) is performed to know platelet count and hematocrit.
c. Blood group is determined prior to platelet collection as group-specific platelet is collected.
d. Across the group platelet collection can also be done with use of platelet additive solutions (PAS) kits.
e. Transfusion-transmitted infection screening is performed prior to collection based on the institutional protocol, whereas in whole blood donation, it is performed after collection.
f. Vein selection is also important so that access pressure could be maintained throughout the procedure.

Troubleshooting steps for different alarms			
S. N.	*Resolution steps for "Draw pressure low"*	*S. N.*	*Resolution steps for "Return pressure high"*
1	Ask the donor to squeeze the handgrip	1	Ask the donor not to squeeze the handgrip
2	Check the BP cuff pressure and increase it up to 40 mm Hg	2	Check the BP cuff pressure and reduce if required
3	Check the needle position and adjust if required	3	Check the needle position and adjust if required
4	Reduce the draw pump speed	4	Reduce the return pump speed
	"Centrifuge pressure high"		*"Pressure test failure"*
1	Stop the centrifuge	1	Check if both the white clamps in the donor line are closed
2	Open the centrifuge door and check if the kit is loaded properly and there are no kinks	2	Check if any tubing is stuck behind the cassette or any obstructions, if so, touch unload, clear the obstruction and then load again
3	Close the door and press continue	3	Check if the pump headers and cassette are loaded correctly
	"Low platelet concentration detected"		*"Leak detected"*
1	Check for the fluid in the plasma and platelet line, if not present, stop the centrifuge and then restart it	1	Stop the centrifuge
		2	Open the centrifuge door
2	Check for platelet clumping and reduce the same (by increasing the AC ratio)	3	Check for any leakage. If any leakage then abort the procedure.
3	Increase the platelet yield	4	If any moisture, clean the leak detector and restart
		5	Touch continue to resume the procedure
	"RBC spillover"		*"Level sensor error"*
1	Increase the HCT by 3% and a maximum up to 9%	1	Check for any air bubbles in the reservoir low-level sensor and TAP the reservoir to clear it

FURTHER READING

1. AABB Technical Manual, 21st Edition, AABB, AABB, Bethesda, MD, 2023.
2. Annual Report 2022. Central Pollution Control Board. https://cpcb.nic.in/status-of-implementation-of-plastic-waste/
3. Annual Report on Biomedical Waste Management for the year 2022 as per Biomedical Waste Management Rules, 2016 by the central pollution control board. Available from: https://cpcb.nic.in/uploads/Projects/Bio-Medical-Waste/AR_BMWM_2022.pdf
4. Facilitator's Guide Ministry of Health anzd Family Welfare Government of India for Blood Bank Lab Technicians & BCSU Medical Officers Training Program. Available from: https://naco.gov.in/sites/default/files/FG_LTs%20BCSU%20DAY%201-5_9%207%202015.pdf
5. Green L, Allard S, Cardigan R. Modern banking, collection, compatibility testing and storage of blood and blood components. Anaesthesia. 2015 Jan;70:3-e2.
6. Harmening DM. Modern blood banking & transfusion practices. FA Davis; 2018 Nov 30.
7. Klein HG, Anstee DJ. Mollison's blood transfusion in clinical medicine. John Wiley & Sons; 2013 Nov 14.
8. RN Makroo. Principles & Practice of Transfusion Medicine 2nd Edition 2018.
9. Rudmann SV. Textbook of blood banking and transfusion medicine. Elsevier Health Sciences; 2005 Feb 18.
10. Simon Toby L, Gehrie Eric A, McCullough Jeffrey, et al. Rossi's Principles of Transfusion Medicine. 6th Ed. John Wiley & Sons, Inc., 111 River Street, Hoboken, NJ 07030, USA.
11. Standards For Blood Banks & Blood Transfusion Services. National AIDS Control Organization. Ministry of Health and Family Welfare. Government of India New Delhi. 2007. Available from: https://naco.gov.in/sites/default/files/Standards%20for%20Blood%20Banks%20and%20Blood%20Transfusion%20Services.pdf
12. Transfusion Medicine Technical Manual. 3rd Ed. NBTC and Blood Transfusion Services Division. Directorate General of Health Services. Ministry of Health & Family Welfare, Government of India. 2023. Available from: https://dghs.gov.in/Uploaddata/Transfusion%20Medicine%20Technical%20Manual%202023.pdf
13. Whitaker B, Rajbhandary S, Kleinman S, Harris A, Kamani N. Trends in United States blood collection and transfusion: results from the 2013 AABB blood collection, utilization, and patient blood management survey. Transfusion. 2016 Sep;56(9):2173–83.
14. World Health Organization. Action framework to advance universal access to safe, effective and quality-assured blood products 2020–2023. World Health Organization; 2020 Mar 16.
15. World Health Organization. Regional Office for the Eastern Mediterranean. (1994). Blood transfusion: a basic text. Available from: https://iris.who.int/handle/10665/119520.

Index